MW01673158

BEYOND THE REFRIGERATOR:

NAVIGATING LIFE AFTER WEIGHT -LOSS SURGERY

LINDA OUELLETTE, LPC

BookLocker
Saint Petersburg, Florida

Print ISBN: 978-1-64719-593-9
Email ISBN: 978-1-64719-594-6

Published by BookLocker.com, Inc., St. Petersburg, Florida.

Printed on acid-free paper.

BookLocker.com, Inc.
2021

First Edition

DISCLAIMER

This book details the author's personal experiences with and opinions about bariatric surgery. The author is not a healthcare provider.

The author and publisher are providing this book and its contents on an “as is” basis and make no representations or warranties of any kind with respect to this book or its contents. The author and publisher disclaim all such representations and warranties, including for example warranties of merchantability and healthcare for a particular purpose. In addition, the author and publisher do not represent or warrant that the information accessible via this book is accurate, complete, or current.

The statements made about eating disorders and bariatric surgery are the author’s personal experience. They are not intended to diagnose, treat, cure, or prevent any condition or disease. Please consult with your own physician or healthcare specialist regarding the suggestions and recommendations made in this book.

Except as specifically stated in this book, neither the author or publisher, nor any authors, contributors, or other representatives will be liable for damages arising out of or in connection with the use of this book. This is a comprehensive limitation of liability that applies to all damages of any kind, including (without limitation) compensatory; direct, indirect, or consequential damages; loss of data, income, or profit; loss of or damage to property and claims of third parties.

You understand that this book is not intended as a substitute for consultation with a licensed healthcare practitioner, such as your physician. Before you begin any healthcare program, or change your lifestyle in any way, you will consult your physician or other licensed healthcare practitioner to ensure that you are in good health and that the examples contained in this book will not harm you.

This book provides content related to topics physical and/or mental health issues. As such, use of this book implies your acceptance of this disclaimer.

TABLE OF CONTENTS

ACKNOWLEDGEMENTS

To the many people who I have encountered and who have helped me along on my journey, I owe you my humblest thanks. I have the greatest respect and the deepest fondness for my former colleague, Del Worley, without whom many things in my abundant life would not have been possible. To my mother, Joy, my thanks for contributing more than you will ever know to my development and my life. To my son, Michael, who quietly supports me in all my endeavors. To my daughter, Julie, who, when I told her of my plans to give up sugar for one month, all too knowingly asked me "Wouldn't you rather give up vegetables instead?" To my dear, sweet husband, Dave, who, for the past 36 years, has tirelessly supported me through all my trials and tribulations, and who is the living embodiment of our vows "for better, for worse, for richer, for poorer, in sickness and in health, as long as we both shall live." And, lastly, to our beloved Labradors, Eclipse and Ruby, who taught me how to swim.

INTRODUCTION

Before bariatric surgery I was 100 pounds overweight, with Type II diabetes, hypertension, and sleep apnea. I "qualified" for weight-loss surgery with a BMI over 35, and co-morbid conditions. These health issues resolved as a result of my weight-loss surgery. From the very first day after my surgery, I have not needed any medication for diabetes or for hypertension. Both of these conditions are within a normal range for me now. My sleep apnea has resolved. Bariatric surgery saved my life.

What bariatric surgery did NOT do was "cure" my desire or need to overeat* and, to be completely honest, I really thought it would. Sure, I went to those support group meetings before my surgery. I heard them say that the surgery was only a tool; that the surgeon was operating on my stomach, not my brain. I smiled and nodded politely but, secretly, I did not believe them. I thought my eating disorder* would be gone after the surgery. (**for the sake of clarity and brevity, and because I view my desire or need to overeat and my obsession with food to exceed what might be considered "normal" I will use the term "eating disorder" to describe my experience with food.)*

I remember a friend who had had the surgery telling me she did not think about food all the time anymore. When she told me that, I thought the surgery would be worth it just for that, even if I never lost any weight. I know now that she was probably one of those unusual overweight people who *did not* have an eating disorder.

I lost 80 pounds in the first eight months after my surgery and then my weight loss leveled off. I did not lose all the weight I wanted to. My eating disorder reminded me of that fact *every day*. I had not gotten down to the weight I wanted to be, the weight my eating disorder wanted me to be. I even began to regain a little weight two years post-surgery, which my surgeon assured me was typical. I kept the 80 pounds off for over a year, but slowly, the compulsive eating returned, and my weight began to inch its way up. They told me that I was going to have to change my lifestyle after the surgery, and I did for a while, a short while. Then old behaviors began to creep back in, as I could get away with them, and, over time, as I could physically eat more, my portions got a bit bigger, and my weight started to increase.

I did not know that my stomach would be able to hold more food over time. I had chosen the vertical sleeve gastrectomy for just that reason. I had heard about the stomach pouch stretching with the gastric bypass and with the adjustable lap band. The sleeve, the surgeon said, was different. Because of the direction of the cut on the stomach, and the fact that one was left with a small cylinder for a stomach rather than a pouch, there was not going to be stretching to worry about. In the very first days after surgery, I could not "eat" much at all. I say "eat" because for the first two weeks my surgeon's food plan limited me to a disgustingly sweet protein drink. In the third week I could add one egg, once a day. To be able to go two whole weeks without food, my eating disorder was in heaven! I would never have made a good anorexic because I love to eat too much. My surgeon told me about how everything was swollen internally at the start, and that I would soon be able to consume more than the initial two ounces that constituted a "meal." My surgery nutritionist had pretty much put the fear of God into all of us and I behaved according to their rules, for a time. I remember the first cracker I had. I felt guilty because it was really the first carbohydrate, I had had in four months, and I knew that crackers were not exactly on the food plan. We were warned about "snacking" and were told to limit ourselves to three small meals a day, with nothing in between. When I ate that first cracker the world did not tumble down around me. I did not become violently ill. The food police did not appear to snatch me away from the jaws of death (well, except maybe in my head!). As time went on, I could gradually eat more food, even well past the time of swelling. I no longer believed the surgeon when he told me my stomach had not stretched. His theory was that the excess food was backing up into my esophagus. Well, whether my stomach had stretched or there was some other explanation, I could certainly eat more at two years post-surgery than I could at a year. And I could eat more at a year than I could at six months.

My eating disorder interpreted all of this as "I am a bad person." I am "bad" because I let old behaviors creep back in. I am "bad" because my weight had gone up. I even wondered if there was a way that I could write this book without mentioning the weight gain. My eating disorder at its best. My eating disorder still tried to convince me that I was hopeless, and I would never change. If that were true, then why not overeat? I wrestled with those beliefs; they were so ingrained.

At two years post-surgery, I had to go back to the idea of changing my lifestyle. Surely, it was not too late! I had not ruined my surgery, or my stomach, or my life! I could learn to deal with this eating disorder, and all the thoughts and feelings that went along with it. FEELINGS??? Ugh! I overate so I would not have to feel feelings. I found that I could no longer avoid them and still maintain my weight. The need for soothing and comfort was what brought me to food in the first place, so awfully long ago. I would learn to get comfort and soothing from other sources. I would learn to talk back to my eating disordered thinking. Working with a nutritionist, I would learn about what foods and portions were right for my "new" body. With a broader understanding of the complexity of what I was dealing with, I embarked on a journey. A journey I will share with you. My husband traveled this journey with me, and you will hear about his experiences as my invaluable support person. Others have traveled this journey as well, and I will share some of their experiences.

I know that I am not alone in my journey. Weight-loss surgery is becoming more popular. Already there are people talking about weight regain after weight-loss surgery. People are talking about the emotional experience of food and understanding that people who have had bariatric surgery are not immune from weight gain and continuing weight struggles. Admitting, though, that the continuing struggle points to an eating disorder is a leap that we seem hesitant to make. The correlation between deciding to have weight-loss surgery and already having an eating disorder needs to be addressed. There are a host of solutions available to people with eating disorders that would assist people who had had weight-loss surgery and are struggling with weight regain. My eating disorder will be with me for the rest of my life. Losing weight changed me externally, but the internal work still needed to be done. I needed to make peace with my eating disorder if I was going to thrive in my new body and enjoy my new life.

MY JOURNEY

It is almost impossible for me to pinpoint the origins of my eating disorder. There are *so* many factors to consider, and they probably all play a role. I think I figured out how to use food for everything *but* nourishment as I grew up. Food has always been love, comfort, soothing, entertainment and FUN for me. With all of the yummy, prepackaged, prefabricated, pre-portioned, instant gratification foods out there, it is a wonder everyone does not have an eating disorder.

My parents struggled with their weight, although their parents did not seem to. I do believe, regardless, that there is a genetic tendency toward a certain body shape and size. There were many diets that my parents tried and, as I became older and more worried about my own weight, I joined right in. I seemed to like the diets that did not restrict quantity. I remember liking one where you could eat as much protein and veggies as you wanted. I also liked a low carbohydrate diet, where you limited your carbohydrate intake to 60 grams a day and ate lots of other stuff. Sixty grams of carbohydrate a day is pretty generous by today's standards, when you look at some of the popular diets out there.

I gained ten pounds a year each year of high school and thought that was normal. I was 150 pounds when I graduated high school in 1975, gained 30 pounds when I quit smoking in 1980, and was 180 pounds when I got married in 1984. I gained 60 pounds with my first pregnancy and 45 pounds with my second. Some of that weight I lost after I delivered, but not a lot. I remember joking that I was "still waiting" to lose the weight I had gained with my second child when she was 14 years old! The day before my bariatric surgery I weighed 242 pounds.

I had only lost weight successfully by dieting a couple of times in my adult life. There was the time that I put myself on a strict 1200 calorie a day diet and counted everything. The problem was I was drinking at the time (I am a recovering alcoholic) and 600 of those 1200 calories had to be for alcohol. At this same time, I was in an aerobics class three times a week, so I did lose weight. During a saner time in my life, I joined a popular weight loss program. I lost 40 pounds in about eight months and kept it off for about 45 seconds. Shortly after I reached my goal weight, I became pregnant and ravenous. I had a miscarriage at ten weeks, but I kept right on eating.

At another time, I discovered a food plan that consisted of no sugar and no flour of any kind, not even the rice flour that is in soy sauce. Grains were allowed - oatmeal, rye, potatoes, barley, etc., just no breads or anything. I followed the plan for three months, and did lose 30 pounds; however, I ate so many baked potatoes in that three months that it was three *years* before I could eat another one. I still think about going back to that weight loss program or the no sugar/no flour plan when I get really desperate. The no sugar/no flour plan comes up when I am feeling like a "bad" person because of how I eat, and somehow, I think following that plan will make me "good" again. I do think that the weight loss program I was in is the safest way to lose weight, but my eating disorder rebels against the limits imposed by any weight loss plan. What usually happens is that I will start to follow a food plan and I will be able to follow it for a few days, or sometimes only for a few hours. Then my eating disorder screams "DEPRIVATION!!!!!" and I start to overeat to compensate. A case in point, as I was writing this chapter, I remembered that I did like one of the diets I was on as a teen, and I decided to try it again. I lasted a day and a half.

I have been in therapy for a long time, and at various intervals have focused on my eating disorder. There were a lot of childhood issues I needed to work through, and I kept thinking that once those were all resolved my eating disorder would no longer be needed and it would fade away. My eating disorder, however, is self-propelled and continues as long as I indulge in it whether there are "reasons" for my overeating or not. Sometimes I think I am ruled by the sheer habit of overeating. Other times I can definitely trace a trigger that started a particular episode. I am almost always trying to avoid feeling some emotion that I suspect will be painful. Avoidance of pain at any cost has been my typical coping style. Food has fit into that quite nicely. It is almost always available, it tastes good, it is soothing and comforting, and it acts as a buffer between my consciousness and whatever feeling it is that I am trying to avoid.

I think that overeating was my first "addiction." Food was important in our household, and restaurant eating in particular made me feel special. When things were chaotic at home, there was respite in a restaurant. I remember a very fancy restaurant in Chicago that was quite a treat when I was a child. I remember the long linen tablecloths and the garlic toast rounds they served in the breadbasket. As I shared this memory with my mother, we were both interested and not too surprised that our memories about places and times often involve food. We remember restaurants that we liked, or even special dishes prepared by our favorite places. What I remember about one of my housekeepers when I was little, besides her girth, is the fact that every Tuesday night, when my mother worked late, she prepared a pan full of fried chicken to cook in the oven. She also made us wonderful lunches. Anything was actually wonderful because our previous housekeeper had only made peanut butter and jelly sandwiches for lunch, every day.

I remember the restaurant that served a generous half chicken dinner on a mound of French fries. I remember my brother's egg roll phase, when we would go to a Chinese restaurant and he would want nothing but egg rolls. That usually started an argument. I remember my grandmother's dry pot roast and the way my other grandmother taught me to eat sunny side up eggs, where first you would cut away all the white and then you would try to scoop it and get the whole yolk into your mouth without breaking it. I still eat my eggs that way.

I do have childhood memories that are not food related, but I believe it is telling that I have so many memories that are. My mother told me that every important decision she and my father made was made over a meal, most often in a restaurant. That was their time when they needed to talk. That held true for my husband and me as well. Some of this, I believe, is inherent in our culture. I do not think my family was that unusual in its focus on food. Food plays a tremendously important role in the American lifestyle. Almost all important celebrations revolve around food. We eat when people are born and we eat when people die, and we eat at every major mile marker in between.

As I said, restaurants were particularly special for me as a child. One very vivid memory I have is the night we were going to go out to a restaurant and my mother and brother were arguing about where we were going to go. We all went downstairs and got into the car, while my mother and brother continued to argue. Finally, my mother had enough and decided that we just were not going to go anywhere. We all went back upstairs and back into the apartment. I had so been looking forward to eating out. My disappointment was overwhelming.

A few years later I remember another night in particular. Very often my mother would "dish on the plates" in the kitchen and present full plates of food to each of us at the table. Well, on this particular night, I was probably 12 or 13 years old, I looked around and noticed that my father got the most amount of food, my brother got the second most amount of food, my mother got the third most amount of food and I got the least. That there was such a noticeable difference in serving sizes is one important point. The fact that I noticed it shows how much I focused on food. How I interpreted it is the most interesting part of the story. I decided that it meant that *men are more important than women.* They had to be more important because they got more food! What I know now is that my mother was often on a diet and that is likely why she had given herself a smaller serving, but I did not know that then.

I cannot tell my story without talking about the other things I did to escape how I was feeling – alcohol and drugs. My first foray into drugs was diet pills. You could get amphetamines right from your family doctor in those days. I remember taking them with the express intention of feeling better. I was not trying to lose weight or lose my appetite; I was trying to lose being depressed. I tried various other drugs off and on throughout high school. Once I understood the potential for weight loss, I eagerly tried amphetamines again, but they made me MORE hungry, not less! For some unknown reason, when I went to college and became of legal drinking age (18 in Wisconsin at that time) I got scruples. I decided I did not want to break the law anymore, so I stopped playing with illicit drugs and just started to drink. A little drinking quickly became a lot of drinking, and I had another escape from the depression that continued to plague me. I do not think they really treated depression in adolescents in those days, so I was pretty much on my own to find a "cure." My obsession with food was definitely quieter when I was drinking. I had found a good numbing agent and used it for several years, until it stopped working. Problem was that alcohol is a *depressant*, so eventually it made me feel worse instead of better. Getting sober was necessary, though not easy. I went to the experts, 12-step programs.

Then my addiction to overeating really began to accelerate. Alcohol is liquid sugar, and I needed to replace the sugar I was not getting any more from the alcohol. After recovery meetings we would go as a group for coffee, and I always had dessert. I expected to lose weight when I quit drinking, I mean, look at all those calories I was not ingesting anymore! I ended up just replacing them with other calories, other sugar. I volunteered in an alcohol treatment center when I had been sober a little while, and for alcohol cravings they would give the patients orange juice *with honey in it*! Talk about sugar!

More serious dieting started. The weight came off. It went back on. Then it came off. Then it went back on. You know the drill. For some reason, the 12-Step principles that were helping me stay sober just did not translate to my food addiction. The most debilitating part of all of this was the shame. Shame that was at my very core. I believed I was "bad" because I could not control how I ate. I was "bad" when I gained weight and "good" when I lost weight. My days were determined by the scale, by how my clothes fit, by whether I exercised. I had to be perfect (more about that later), and nowhere was that more evident than with my food. If I was following a diet, I had to do it perfectly. What I loved most about the popular weight loss program was that I got a brand new, blank food journal every Monday, and all the imperfections of the previous week were gone! This week I would do better! This week I would be perfect! I kept all those food journals, and when I reached goal, I went back over them and counted the days I had been "on program" and the days I had been off. I had been "off program" about 1/3rd of the time. Definitely NOT perfect, but I had reached goal weight anyway. I went through six weeks of their Maintenance program, gradually adding calories to my daily total to see where my weight would level off. At the end of the six weeks, I was up to adding 450 calories a day to their program. That is a whole piece of pie! Dessert became my dearest friend, again.

Fast forward 25 years… Life… Children - 2… Careers - 3… Alcohol relapse and getting sober again… Eating Disorder treatment… Dieting… Losing weight… Gaining weight… Memories surfacing from times forgotten in childhood… Therapy and more therapy… Graduate school… Becoming a counselor to help others as I recovered from my own struggles… More therapy. Persistently struggling with my eating, my food, my weight, and the nagging shame. No matter what I tried, I just could not seem to get a handle on my eating disorder. Full blown by this point, there was no mistaking it. I lived, breathed, and existed for food, mostly sugar. I had always wanted to be bulimic but could never manage to intentionally vomit. I was too food obsessed to be anorexic. I did not binge like you see those teenage girls do in those ABC afterschool specials on TV. I just overate consistently and constantly. I simply could not stop.

I tried everything, including trying nothing. I got to a point where the mere thought of a diet was enough to trigger the deprivation monster and cause me to overeat. "Abstinence" for me became NOT trying to do anything about my weight or my eating. I had become so crazy with this diet, or that exercise plan that I had to "abstain" from all of that insanity. My eating disorder was in heaven! I had finally given up and stopped trying to control it. Sanity became defined as not fighting my eating disorder- but in not fighting, I was losing. The days when I ate what I wanted, when I wanted and did not struggle *seemed* peaceful. At least the shame was quiet. I did have days where I felt OK about how I looked, about how I ate. I was not actually looking or eating any differently, I was just not beating myself up over it. The shame was the killer, because I had to keep overeating to get rid of that awful feeling, that hating myself to my very core. The shame fueled a lot of the eating disorder, but even when the shame was quiet, the eating disorder persisted. This puzzled both my therapist and me, as it was quite clear that overeating produced shame which produced more overeating. Get rid of the shame, we figured, and we would have half the cycle eliminated. There was still the overeating, however, at the beginning of the cycle. Anything might trigger that. I would overeat to escape painful or uncomfortable feelings. I would overeat because they played a pizza commercial at 5:30pm before I had started making dinner. I would overeat on Tuesday when they had aired that pizza commercial on Monday. I had cravings and obsessions that did not quit until I satisfied them. Once I had a food thought in my head it lived there, at full volume most of the time, until I did something about it. I was easily influenced by the media. We all are. Billboards, commercials, slogans, jingles. Let us face it - advertising works!

Sometimes I could easily trace the trigger for a particular bout of overeating. Other times it was a mystery. Painstakingly, I would try and rewind the tape and trace the overeating back to its source. Perhaps I had become uncomfortable with a coworker three days ago. Maybe my husband had said something to one of our children that upset me. Or something had come up in therapy that I was struggling with. Sometimes I could not come up with a clear trigger at all, no matter how hard I tried or where I searched. The real puzzlers turned out to be the ones that *looked* like they were food related triggers, which were really emotional triggers in disguise. Maybe I would have that pizza on Tuesday, after that commercial on Monday, but then that was not enough and I had to eat a large dessert after that, and maybe go out for breakfast the next morning. All of a sudden, the shame was back, and I was mired in it. *Then* I might remember a disagreement I had had with someone several days earlier. Or perhaps I had not spoken up for myself with someone when I wanted something a particular way, or I had been hurt by something that had happened.

It took a long time for me to even see, or admit, that there were emotional triggers for my eating disorder. The idea of powerlessness needs to be mentioned here. Twelve-step programs are based on the premise that there is a disease process in play, and that the person is powerless over the management of that disease process. I have never made peace with that concept. First of all, if I am powerless, then I am not "bad" like my shame tells me I am. Some people might be relieved at that, but my shame is so entrenched that it does not want to let go. Secondly, and in contrast, as I search for triggers for the overeating, I find that I play more of an active role in the whole eating disorder than the concept of powerlessness allows for. One school of thought believes that there is a large physical role that food plays in eating disorders and believes it is important to abstain from one's trigger foods, especially common ones like white flour or sugar. Another school of thought is that it is not about the food at all, and that all foods are allowed. I have always leaned more towards the second school of thought. I do believe that, for me at least, overeating is much more about emotions than it is about physiology, and as I have learned to deal more effectively with emotional issues, I have had quieter times with my eating disorder.

I find it interesting to ponder about my weight-loss surgery and how that figures into my eating disorder. As I discussed the possibility of weight-loss surgery in therapy, the therapist I was seeing at the time cautioned me that wanting the surgery was a symptom of the eating disorder and would not resolve those issues for me. Of course, I did not believe her. The weight-loss surgery would be THE answer, the cure, the end to the eating disorder. This therapist, it turns out, was partly right. I had health issues involved with my obesity that "resolved" (the medical term the doctors use) with the surgery. I must confess however that, as virtuous as it appears, I did not have the surgery to take care of these health issues. I had the surgery to look better, to feel better about myself, and to END my eating disorder. The fact that it would improve my health was secretly inconsequential. I had resigned myself to living with these health issues and if they would shorten my life, then so be it. They seemed to be fairly well controlled by medications, and I had good health insurance, so the costs were manageable. Related to this discussion is the fact that my father died of esophageal cancer at the age of 73. My mother asked him, when he was near the end, if he wished he had eaten differently and dealt with his own obesity so he would have lived longer. His answer was "No." Facing death perhaps ten years earlier than if he had not been obese, he would not have changed his penchant for overeating. It turns out that esophageal cancer is related to obesity, as was his high blood pressure, his diabetes, and his sleep apnea.

My surgery journey began with an informational meeting where I learned about the different types of bariatric surgery. I decided on the vertical sleeve gastrectomy. This procedure was still considered "experimental," having only been around for about seven years, thus, my insurance would not cover the cost. I chose this procedure regardless primarily for the reason that there was not supposed to be a risk of the stomach stretching if one ate too much. With the gastric bypass I was concerned about the malabsorption of nutrients and "dumping syndrome." Dumping syndrome refers to food and gastric juices from your stomach moving to your small intestine in an unregulated, abnormally fast manner. Symptoms are flu-like.

Approximately one third to one half of gastric bypass surgery patients will develop at least mild dumping syndrome (www.Mayoclinic.com). It is most likely to occur after eating larger amounts of sugar. Thus, if I were to have the gastric bypass, I would get sick if I ate a lot of sugar. The bariatric surgeons, probably none of whom have eating disorders, believe that this dumping syndrome is a tool that acts as a deterrent to eating a lot of sugar. In my disease, I was quite sure I would not be able or willing to give up sugar, and I was afraid that I would eat it anyway, and then pay the consequences.

In researching the Lap Band, I discovered that the average maintained weight loss after surgery was approximately 40% of one's excess weight. Well, 40% was not near enough for me! Why go through all the pain and expense of the surgery to lose only 40% of what I wanted to lose?

The vertical sleeve resembles the old stomach stapling but is much more effective. The surgeon, most often laparoscopically, pinches off a large portion of the stomach vertically. The 85% of your stomach that will no longer be involved in the digestive process is actually removed from your body. The result is that your stomach now is more like a conduit than a reservoir. The regular digestion process is undisturbed. The valves at both the upper and lower parts of the stomach still function normally. There is no resection or removal of the intestine. Because the stomach is now like a small, narrow tube, instead of a pouch as with the other surgeries, there is not supposed to be stretching to worry about. I would be forever limited in the amount of food I could hold. “Forever!” That is an eating disorder belief, if I have ever heard one.

What was actually my experience is that I was gradually able to eat larger quantities of food, which I believe contributed to my weight regain. I expected to maintain eating the amount of food that I could eat at about six months post-surgery. What happened, in contrast, is that at one year I could eat a little less than twice the amount of food I could eat at six months, and now, at two years plus, I can eat even more than that. Now, you might think that just because I *can*, does not mean I *should,* and you would be right. My eating disorder, however, is most satisfied when I am either binging or restricting, binging being the more likely of the two. Now, I use the word “binge” very generally, as I could not eat as much food at one time as a true binge would be for a compulsive eater. I did eat compulsively, though, often eating past the point of what I would have preferred. I ate for emotional numbing, for comfort, and also for entertainment. At my two-year post-surgery checkup, I asked my surgeon why I could eat so much more food now than before. He said that he did not think my stomach had stretched, but rather believed that the food was backing up into my esophagus. That made some sense based on how I felt when I overate. My shame wanted me to believe that I had stretched out my stomach, that I had been “bad,” and that the weight regain was my “punishment.” My surgeon also said that a mild weight regain is quite common, especially around the time that I was post-surgery. He applauded me for being aware and for wanting to do something about it.

Two other things happened right after surgery that are worth noting. First, I was HUNGRY! They *promised* me I would not be hungry. The literature told me that the portion of my stomach that had been removed was where the hormone ghrelin was made. Ghrelin controls your appetite. So, most people do not experience hunger after their surgery, until several months later when the hunger returns. I was hungry from the very beginning. I could literally feel the emptiness of my stomach. Drinking a protein syrup several times a day, I ate no food, except an occasional jello or broth, for two weeks. Then on week three, in addition to the protein syrup, I could eat one egg every day. The doctors seem to have relaxed this strenuous food plan a bit, as a friend of mine just went through surgery and she was starting solid food before the first week was up. Soft proteins were added gradually, then firmer proteins, then hard proteins. Fruits and vegetables came much later. Starches even later than that.

The second thing to note is that because I was hungry, and because I had an eating disorder, I found it quite difficult not to eat past the point of fullness. Physically, I became excruciatingly uncomfortable when this would happen. Then one day, out of desperation, I tried to make myself throw up. Well, it worked. I continued this practice well into my second-year post-surgery, several times a week at first, then tapering finally to less than a couple of times a month. I was almost always vomiting only to relieve physical discomfort, though I did cross the line at times and overeat something I wanted because I knew I could throw it up right after. Over time, as I became able to eat more food, the physical need for the vomiting decreased. I would get to that feeling of over-fullness much less often, even though I was eating more. My eating disorder saw this as more "evidence" that I was "bad," and I often feared that I would regain all the weight I had lost. Surely, it was only a matter of time.

I found it difficult at first to figure out when to stop eating. The line between enough food and too much was often only one bite different. This bite I would still be fine and then one more bite and I would be uncomfortably full. My stomach was very unforgiving in that regard. I was afraid to not eat enough food. Surely this tiny amount would not nourish me! My deprivation alarms went off and I worried about everything. I worried about not eating enough and I worried about eating too much. I worried when I lost weight quickly and when I lost more slowly. I was getting a lot of comments from the people around me. I told most of the people I came into contact with about the surgery. I wanted them to understand what I was doing that was so successful. I wanted them to know what I had gone through, and not just think it was "magic." People, in general, were amazed and very complimentary. There was a certain "high" to the period of rapid weight loss. I lost 30 lbs. in the first three weeks. Once I was a way out from my surgery, and a couple of people I knew were just having surgery, I envied them their "honeymoon period," remembering how wonderful I felt in those first few months. And now that I had regained a small amount of the weight I had lost, surely, I could find a way back to that honeymoon period. Surely, I could replicate that food plan and start losing again. At that time, I was doing two protein shakes a day and one small meal. I could do that again, couldn't I? I found that I could not. My eating disorder, now used to eating more food again, would not sacrifice one morsel of food in the interest of weight loss. My eating disorder spoke to me, assuring me that I would eventually regain all the weight I had lost and that I might as well just give in and let it win. It told me my life would be so much more peaceful if I did not struggle with it, and just gave it what it wanted. I had to find a way to master this dysfunctional, sabotaging thinking, or it would be right!

I dealt with my eating disorder issues in individual therapy, and in a women's group for people with eating disorders. The group was helpful in terms of knowing that I was not alone in my struggles. Lots of women grapple with food/weight/body image issues, whether they have eating disorders or not. My discussions, however, seemed to be mostly about symptoms and not about recovery. I would report in that I had had a "good" week when I felt like I had control of my overeating and maybe had even lost weight. "Bad" weeks were times when I felt out of control, and my weight was inching up. Those two words – "good" and "bad" - were attached to everything I did in terms of my food. I could not eliminate them from my vocabulary! Yet, I had a sense that I would feel a lot more peace in my life if I could. I read books. I went to workshops. I did everything I could think of to find that magic answer to stop regaining weight. There were a lot of things that helped, albeit temporarily. Maybe the trick was to string a lot of those temporary helps together over time. Maybe today it would help to talk to a friend when I wanted to overeat, yet tomorrow I would need to do something different. This went against the "black and white" thinking of my eating disorder, which told me there was ONE answer to my problem and I just had not found it yet. Perhaps there were several answers, each that would work in its own time. I knew that "recovery" was not going to be about the food, for me. I knew it had to do with facing those day-to-day feelings and stressors that I did not want to face. It had to do with not numbing myself with a carbohydrate haze. I used to think that some deep, dark buried trauma was fueling the eating disorder, and once I discovered it, the eating disorder would fade away. With all the work I had done in therapy, however, I no longer thought there was any deep, dark buried anything. I had remembered disturbing events, and dealt with those feelings and processed them, and still I overate. I was doing so much better now. I was so much healthier and happier. Surely, I could stop the overeating now? Nope. It was not buried trauma that made me eat. It was being unable (or unwilling?) to deal with the everyday stress of "life on life's terms," as they say. I ate to relieve stressful feelings, and then got stuck in the guilt and shame about overeating. I had a running dialogue with my eating disorder all day long.

[Eating disorder] "Eat this. You'll feel better."

[Me] "I'd really rather not."

[Eating disorder] "Oh, come on, you know you want it. Just have one."

[Me] "Oh, ok. I guess this time it might be different. Maybe I can have just one."

Then, once I overate, having several more than just one, the dialogue became:

[Eating disorder] "Well, you overdid it again. You better not eat the rest of the day to make up for it. You'd better sign up for that weight loss program again because you will never do this on your own. You're too weak."

[Me] "You're right. I am bad. I am out of control. I will use your idea of restricting to get back in control. Next time it will be different."

And there was always a next time, often even the same day.

So, there was my eating disorder doing a complete flip on me! No wonder I was so confused. First it would entice me to overeat, and then it would tell me to restrict to make up for it. First it wanted me out of control and then it wanted to punish me for being so! I could not win! And, if I engaged in this dialogue, back and forth, all day long, I never dealt with the stressful feelings that had come up to begin with! I was trapped in an endless loop.

How could I get out of this trap, this seemingly endless loop? I tried a lot of things. Some things helped, some things did not. I will share these with you. There was a connection between my having an eating disorder and my having had weight-loss surgery. I got to the point of needing the weight-loss surgery *because* I had an eating disorder. The eating disorder was there from a noticeably young age. Perhaps your weight issues come from a younger time in your life. Perhaps not. There might be suggestions here that will work for you. There are coping tools that people with eating disorders have been using for a long time. These tools can enter the world of bariatric surgery. They need to. If we are to survive our surgery, overcome the eating disorder and go on to live happy, sane lives, we need tools that work.

MY HUSBAND'S JOURNEY

ABOUT ME

It may be helpful to first discuss my own background in the context relevant to this book. It will not take awfully long: middle age, average height, and average weight. Whether I would be classified a liberal conservative, or a conservative liberal is a debatable point that will keep my family entertained for years ahead. Suffice it to say I work hard trying to keep an open mind, even when that may not be my first inclination. I do prefer to think my way through things, which is in keeping with my engineering and science background. The words, "spontaneous" and "impulsive" are unlikely to be engraved on my headstone. Doctors, dentists, and psychologists will not see me as a patient until it is nearly too late. Trends and fads hold no interest for me. I cannot recall what I had for dinner two nights ago. I have never been on a diet. At least, I do not think I have been, but I will explore that later.

Early in my twenties, I participated in an anonymous, self-help group for those afflicted by the effects of another's compulsions or addictions. I am eternally grateful to that entity and to those individuals: I thank you sincerely. Through my decade with them I learned a small set of tools that I would use throughout my adulthood. It helped me to be a better husband, and a better parent. Perhaps I did not follow all the suggestions by the book, so to speak. But armed with the tools of detachment, acceptance, and self-assessment, I felt capable of embracing life's challenges. I always knew where to go for a "personal tune-up" if I needed it, and there was comfort in that knowledge. My coping tools may have virtual rust marks and signs of wear and tear, but like my favorite screwdriver and wrench, they work just as well as when shiny and new. They are comfortable in my hand, and I know what to expect of them.

As for labels, I do not like them very much. They are unimpressive on clothing; they are uninteresting on food; and frankly, they do not suit people very well at all. Yet if you are compelled to hang "codependent" on me, I will not argue vehemently—so long as it makes you happy. That is about it.

CONTEMPLATING

The discussion of surgical weight loss came as no surprise. There was a sudden flood of billboard and radio advertisements in town promoting surgical solutions, and my inner voice said the topic would come soon. I waited. Surprisingly, I waited more. The topic finally surfaced later than I had expected; however, the amount of research she had done explained the apparent delay.

There was a clarity and certainty in her procedure selection that was unmistakable. A calm, detached assessment of why the vertical sleeve gastrectomy was the proper choice over other available options. And there was a palpable sense of finality: this was it. Now my fear rose. There was no real fear about the surgery or recovery itself, aside from the normal concerns. I did worry what would happen if/when this surgery turns out not to be the answer? Part of me wished she had decided on the Lap-Band alternative just so that there would still be an available option further down the road. Another part of me was secretly relieved, for I had envisioned countless trips to the doctor to adjust the mechanism. At least with most of the stomach gone, cause-and-effect would be easier. I naively thought that eliminating much of the stomach would also eliminate worrying about the organ once surgical recovery was complete.

The finality of removing 85% of one's stomach brought me now to a new understanding. After all these years, I was just now beginning to gain some insight into her desperation. Eating disorders kill—I knew that in my head, but now it had reached my heart.

PRE-SURGERY

I attended several of the weekly support meetings before the surgery. The meetings consisted of a large group of people who were considering various surgical electives; patients getting ready for upcoming surgery; patients who recently had a procedure; and family members. Here I met the surgeon and some of the staff. Meeting them was extremely helpful to me, and I felt confident in their experience. The meetings themselves were a bit surreal to me. There were tables with various dietary supplement products available, along with some samples. It made sense that patients should have an opportunity to try some of the foods they would be eating before and after surgery, but it caught me by surprise. I do not connect "hospitals" with "marketing" in my mind. I noticed some staff members were sporting large picture buttons with their pre-surgery photos. Though I am not a big fan of such things, the pride they had in changing their lives was apparent and powerful. I listened intently when they shared their stories, not so much to the number of pounds lost, but to the impressive health benefits they experienced. The health rewards seemed a common and concrete point. I thought that diabetes reduction and avoiding a future of joint pain were extraordinary benefits of the surgery, regardless of whether the future weight reduction goal number would be achievable.

SURGERY DAY

The medical team impressed me. I trusted the surgeon was top-notch, and knew he had many satisfied clients. He seemed to know Linda very well and seemed genuinely interested in discussing any concerns. I expect doctors to have good bed-side manner, but he was way above the bar in my book. The person I was anxious to meet was the anesthesiologist. In my view, they work the balancing act between life and death, and I have a profound respect for their profession. Unlike her surgeon, the anesthesiologist did not have the advantage of a few pre-surgery appointments to get to know her. I really have no idea how to assess an anesthesiologist, but he seemed sharp, attentive, and intently focused on her. I was happy. It was worth getting up before dawn to be one of the first customers of the day, especially since no one was behind schedule yet.

We had a nurse at the beginning who kept talking on and on about cheesecake. Talk of cheesecake that she had a few days ago; cheesecake that her sister makes; and favorite cheesecake recipes. I doubt the nurse really understood what was ahead for us, or the road behind us. It was nervous chatter from both parties. News from the operating room came in a timely manner. The doctor explained that everything went very well.

The hospital room had a large recliner, where I sat passing time. Given the choice of the bed or the recliner, there was no doubt in my mind I had the most comfortable seat. Since I like technology so much, the pressurized booties on her legs were a constant source of amusement. Pfffft…the left would inflate while the right deflated Pfffft again, and the cycle alternated. I knew these were to reduce the risk of clotting, and the nursing staff was clear about how important they were. Well, at least the first nurse was clear. At the change of shifts, we had new attendants, and it seemed they were slightly less obsessed. Although I do not advocate well for myself, I can be a bulldog for those around me. *Excuse me nurse, aren't those things supposed to be on now?* Challenging medical authority and advocating for patient care was unfamiliar to me. After all, they know best, right? When a meal tray arrived with food that was inappropriate for someone who had just had their stomach altered, my suspicion that even the best care had some glitches was confirmed.

I stayed in the room the first night. Our nurse had instructed us to take a short walk every two hours once she had been examined by the doctor. We agreed, we would walk every two hours throughout the night. I set my watch and we began our strolls as appointed. The first one was difficult, but every time we went there was marked improvement. The evening came to a draw, and we went to sleep. This is to say, I went to sleep in the comfortable recliner, while she tried to sleep in the uncomfortable hospital bed. If that was not bad enough, there was the constant parade of nursing staff with pills and pokes to deal with throughout the night. Midnight: time for a walk. We arose and made another circuit around the ward, wheeling the IV stand to which she was precariously attached and shuffling in those bright yellow non-slip socks they give you. Back "home" again we went back to bed.

Two o'clock was an instant replay. Bzzzz. My watch alarm went off again at 4:00 AM. "Honey, it's time for a walk… Time to get up… Linda?" The response was clear: leave me alone! I was simply happy there was a response, having already imagined horrible things had happened while I slept through them. She was exhausted. I reminded her of the risks that the walks were intended to minimize and how her overall recovery would benefit. Where exactly was I willing to draw the line? How hard would I push, and how compassionate would I be? I decided to relay the facts again, remind her of what we had agreed to ahead of time, and abide by her decision. She bargained to skip this time and promised to do the next. I think the actual words were," …let me sleep now and I won't divorce you..." In any event, it looked like this walk simply was not going to happen. I turned on my side in the darkness. Then she said, "Ok, let's go." We were up and, on our way, strolling the hall – still married.

HOME

As one who does not have a lot of personal, first-hand experience with surgery, there are little details that I forget. The pre-surgery information was well done, and I felt confident enough in my knowledge of incisions, drainage, signs of infection, limits on activity and so forth. But there was one item that totally escaped me: post-surgery nausea.

The initial nausea reaction to the anesthesia was addressed during the recovery phase immediately following the surgery. Management continued throughout the hospital stay but had not fully resolved even when discharge orders were given, so nausea continued to be a concern into the home stay. My worry was simple, perhaps even child-like: can a new, surgically altered stomach withstand all the physical exertion experienced during vomiting? Was there a risk to the "sealed seams" of the stomach? In short, was developing a leak at all probable? How would I know—what would the signs of any internal problems be? My trusty internet searches yielded no information on this topic. I felt alone.

I slept lightly those first few nights. Any trips she made to the bathroom in the middle of the night would be queried with, "Is everything OK?" That was convenient shorthand for, "Did you vomit? Do you have a fever? Extraordinary abdominal pain? Do you think your stomach is OK? Are you worried as much as I am??" I trusted she was going through her own checklist on a routine basis and tried to set aside the possibility that I may be wrong. It was hard to strike a balance between vigilance and meddling. I believed a good mental attitude on her part was an important ingredient to a successful recovery, and I tried to behave accordingly. Consequently, I consciously interpreted every terse "yup" as an expedient, "Everything is A-OK," instead of shorthand for, "Leave me alone." There is power in choosing how you hear things.

The nausea resolved itself after about two days at home, four days post-op. I felt relieved as things seemed to assume a more textbook progression. I was sleeping better, though sadly my partner was now having a bit more difficulty. The fatigue was lessening, but the discomfort seemed to be on the rise. Finding a comfortable sleeping position was a challenge.

I admit to being curious about the surgery sites and was confident that in good time they would be shown to me. I knew and respected the boundaries in this area. The abdomen is an area I feel is designated as off-limits to touch and general discussion. I do not initiate discussions about it even today, regardless of how matter of fact and analytical the topic can be approached. So, the words, "Honey, can I see your belly scars?" were not going to come from my lips. In time they may be shown to me, and I would be honored to be invited into that part of her life. It would wait. And in time, they were revealed. Clean, healthy, and healed, they appeared to be perhaps one-half inch long in various strategic locations. I was amazed at how small these 5 or so incisions were. I was hugely impressed by how "minimally invasive" this operation was. It was a remarkable triumph of medical technology. Yet, it also struck me just how much damage one can do with so little outward sign. It seemed rather bizarre – unfair perhaps – that 85% of the stomach could be removed so quickly and extracted through such small incisions. In my head this operation was a big deal to me, not only because of the physiological aspects, but because of what ultimately was at stake in the long-term. The external evidence did not seem to match the gravity I felt it deserved. And then, I thought how fitting it was that the "insides did not match the outsides." In my own mind, bariatric surgery became its own metaphor for disordered eating. The irony seemed fitting.

EARLY RECOVERY

Weeks two through four after surgery seemed to go as expected for the physical recovery. The operation sites healed pretty much on schedule. The fatigue of the first week was starting to lift, and activities were resuming. Keeping the cat off her stomach when we sat on the couch became a bit of a sport, although it was not quite clear who was winning. I never noticed how many times the cat jumped up on us until *after* surgery. I think our cat exceeded the weight restrictions imposed on post-surgery activity, or perhaps I just took some pleasure in tossing him onto the floor. In any event, the cat was not one of those things I had anticipated.

Weight lifting restrictions are funny things, and I find few people are good judges of how heavy something is as they hold it in their hand. They underestimate. Of course, I tend to be over-protective, so this has great potential for conflict. I wanted to lift everything in sight for her, while she obviously was not interested in being treated as incapable. It did not become a real problem because we came to a verbal agreement early on. I learned to ask first if she wanted help; and she too learned to ask if she experienced any straining in her attempts to lift something. That was basic stuff, but actually saying it and agreeing to it opened up a lot of freedom. I would not hover over her because I knew she would ask, and she could ask me without worry of imposition. No magic here, just Communication 101.

In week two we were beginning to resume life as usual. I had returned to work. My mother-in-law was able to spend some days at the house with her to help. Our daughter was continuing her high school activities in full swing. Our son was conveniently tucked away at the local university. I am sure he is grateful for this. Other than knowing that mom was ok, he did not desire much information. Linda's activity level was coming along quite nicely. We were ready to confront our first big challenge: the family dinner.

In the first week post-op, having meals together was easy to avoid. Linda would eat off-schedule, as necessary. Meanwhile, I would fend for myself as unobtrusively as possible. Our daughter would grab meals out with her friends. With the fatigue she experienced in the first week and need for rest, this worked out relatively well. In the second week and thereafter, this would not work out quite so easily. We were a "dinner together" sort of family.

Once again, we discussed who would cook, what "dinner together" might be like, and what worried us. To her credit, Linda embraced the idea of cooking early on, even though she would not be eating any of the food herself. As she stated it, this was something she had chosen, and she would not go through life without cooking. She liked that role in the family and was going to resume it – modified, perhaps- as well and as soon as possible. We would share cooking, as we did throughout our relationship (though she cooks more than I) and work together on planning. The *experience* of cooking became the bigger picture, and even the most basic meals had something that enhanced their appearance and presentation. She may not be able to taste the food, but sight, sounds, and smells were becoming other aspects to appreciate.

Pork chops were my downfall. Pork chops are a personal favorite of mine, and there is truly little that can be done to ruin one unless you omit the bone. Take a bone-in chop, sear it and pan fry, it does not matter if it is thick or thin, moist, and tender or dry and crunchy, I'm a happy camper. I like to hear them sizzle, smell them in the pan, and gnaw the black crunchies off the bones. I sat at the table that evening with pork chops on my plate. Next to me, she sat with her plastic tube of flavored gelatinous goo. My mind scrambled as we ate, going through my virtual toolkit… here is my detachment tool… aha, I did not cause this, ok…where was my acceptance doohickey thingy? Gotta be around someplace.... As many coping tools as I could conjure up, as quickly as I could do it, I was under siege by guilt. I wanted to cry that night, and frankly, to this day I still do whenever I think on it. I felt guilty about eating a pork chop.

Feeling guilty was second nature to me. My (then future) mother-in-law labeled me as "the department of regret and remorse," as much in jest as in truth. Rightfully so, I think. But I had never experienced guilt regarding food, not like this. Oh, perhaps I experienced some regret in sneaking a cookie before dinner or chocolate during Lent, but this pork chop episode was in a whole league by itself.

There was an audio tape I had listened to many years before that had a wonderful piece on guilt. I cannot find it now, so can only paraphrase what I got out of it, mindful that there is frequently a difference between what was heard, and what was said. The speaker was discussing the function of guilt. I had never before considered that guilt may have a function, but just rather considered it one of those things we carried with us—a sort of psychological appendix. The speaker continued that (my words here) guilt helps us to maintain a self-image of who we are in the presence of behavioral evidence that runs against that image. Simply put, I maintain that I am an honest person. If I act in a manner that runs counter to that, for instance by stealing pens from work, then I feel guilty about that because it runs against my self-image of how an honest person behaves. To resolve the guilt, I either need to change my image of how an honest person behaves (which is hard to do) or change the behavior and stop taking pens home. Following the path of least resistance, I stop walking off with pens and become realigned with my "honest self." At least, that was the understanding I took away from listening to the tape.

I knew I would have to examine this "pork chop guilt." I was fighting the tide of how "good people" should behave regarding food. It is impolite to start eating before everyone around you is served. Eat what is on your plate. Taking second helpings is acceptable only if there is enough for all. Never take the last helping but save it for someone else. And of course, providers do not let their families go hungry. Nor children in foreign nations either, for that matter.

It became clearer to me that I would not be able let go of this struggle. I was having more and more difficulty eating cooked meals while she was on a liquid diet. Though we discussed the ins and outs of this with as much honesty possible, my belief was that when I ate along with her, it bothered her. And I did not want to be the one "bothering" her. Good people do not eat in front of hungry people.

True to form, if I could not change my image of how good people behave-- to accept that they may in fact continue to eat normally in this circumstance-- I would alter my behavior to reduce the guilt load. Some of these alterations were healthy, some not. Eating lunch at work grew to having a large meal then and a smaller dinner. Treats or snacks would be done at lunch, avoiding the evening trap. There were a few instances where we all agreed ahead of time to schedule when our daughter and I would go out for dinner by ourselves. This would later evolve into a ritual father-daughter Saturday lunch at the sub shop while mom was busy at work.

Linda returned to work in the fourth week. It was manageable, but perhaps another week would have suited her better physically. We had taken some test drives in the car together to see how it felt. Was there discomfort if a quick driving maneuver was necessary? Any troubles slamming on the brake? The seatbelt seemed ok, but I was concerned about what the possible consequences would be if the air bag was deployed during an accident. Nevertheless, life moves forward, and you take your chances. Emotionally, getting back into a routine as soon as possible seemed appropriate.

Much of the home routine would involve the groceries. First, there was the planning for the week. With an active teenager in the house, this became a bit challenging despite the absolute best plans. Cooking was touchy enough but adding the last-minute uncertainties of cooking for one or for two (or even three, when her boyfriend came over!) and it became a source of frustration. I could see our daughter grappling with wanting to go out with her friends for dinner while simultaneously wanting to be home with us as a family. She was struggling to find her way. I was worried.

Second, actually making the list was a muddy task. *What sounds good for dinner this week?* Really? I would prefer <u>not</u> to think about it. Under normal circumstances I do not mind too much coming up with a sufficient, though perhaps uninspired list. Chicken, shrimp, fish, a turkey sausage of sorts, and maybe beef… But I was not working under normal circumstances. One thing was certain: pork chops were definitely not going on that list! My idea of helping to make the list became an exercise in trying to identify things that would lack appeal for one reason or another. Shrimp are too pokey and should not be too tempting… Chicken breast can be sufficiently boring if cooked stove-top without any sort of sauces… And that was how I started to analyze cooking options during early recovery.

A trip to the grocery store was the third piece of this puzzle. In this fourth week we would trek to the store together, although not for the first time. We had made an excursion to the store a few times in the preceding weeks to pick up a few items, but it was really more a matter of getting out of the house and changing the scenery. Now we were really in for shopping together. I was concerned over how she might react in the grocery store, if the endless aisles of food possibilities would overwhelm, tempt, or lead to depression. My concern seemed unfounded and shopping itself did not seem to be problematic for her. In truth, it likely had more of an impact on me. I became much more aware of the bakery treats thrust out there; the ever-present ladies with toothpick-laden trays handing out samples, who cannot seem to take no for an answer; the point-of-sale displays stacked in the aisles that must be modeled after road construction barricades. I became agitated with the grocery store and voiced my opinion on a few occasions. Of course, the store had not really changed that much in a month's time, but I was seeing it through new eyes. I was imagining how she might be seeing it. On occasion, the cart may have bumped a display here or there, not to any great damage but to some personal satisfaction. I knew in my heart that food was not the enemy, but I was not so convinced about its marketing anymore.

Aside from some bad cart handling, I mostly served two functions here. These were to retrieve objects that were too high to stretch for, too low to bend for, or too heavy to get into the cart. The second was just to help us stick with the items we had put on the list, which was our agreed plan. We tried to make a list as specific as possible. Listing "chuck roast" instead of "beef" made us focus on exactly what we were after. We did not have to paw over what looked good, or what was on special. It helped me stay on track with my thinking and buying.

Soon, when the list did not include heavy items, she would go shopping by herself. This was a particularly good thing. Women have been going to market without husbands for ages, and perhaps it is the true pillar of marriage. Everyone needs a break now and then, and I certainly did not want to stop her from taking hers.

LATER RECOVERY

I cannot recall when in time the next phase started, only with what. It started with a soft-boiled egg. She had made it through a long series of liquid meals and finally reached the point of limited semi-solid food in her recovery. "I never knew an egg could taste so good," she said. I felt happy for her. I felt happy for her, for me, and for us. I was not willing to predict the future, but it seemed now that there was some light on the path we were walking. There was hope that something resembling "normal" would return. Hope? Normal? Was I feeling hopeless? What did I mean by normal? Huh-what??

The egg triggered something in me, some things I did not realize. One was that by this time, I was beginning to resign myself. That is not a typographic error. In case the spell-checking software alters my sentence during printing, I will restate the sentence with an underscore in place. I was beginning to resign myself. This was not any form of acceptance or healing. Quite the contrary, I was starting an active forfeiture of my personal eating wants and habits. I do not have many food wants. Ask me what I want for dinner or breakfast, and most of the time I will reply, "I don't care." This is true, although it is not particularly helpful. It takes effort for me to stop and think if I am having any particular wants, to get in touch with something to which I am not normally tuned in. I certainly like my lobsters and clams, my chocolate cake, pizza, barbeque chips, and yes, my pork chops. But if you ask me what I want, my face and mind will go blank. So, I began to consider what life might be like without lobster and pizza and started casting them aside. It was just easier to succumb than to fight, to accept an imagined future of separate meals and pureed foods. I chuckled at the thought of sitting alongside her in beach chairs, sporting large straw hats and sunglasses, the waves crashing distantly as we toasted our golden years holding plastic tubes of gelatinous goo adorned with tiny paper umbrellas. I even pondered trying one of the gooey things myself. That is when I knew for sure I was in trouble.

In some situations, one can coast along by not engaging in the same behavior as the afflicted person. Say for discussion's sake that your partner is afflicted with an addiction to lilac flowers. As they go through their struggles with their lilac addiction, you may choose to avoid lilacs altogether. Do not bring lilacs home. Do not use lilac air fresheners. Do not buy lilac perfumes and so on. And if you are rather neutral to lilacs yourself, then avoiding lilacs as a way of life can be very functional. However, I could not avoid food altogether. It is as much a necessity for me as it is for her. The lilac analogy just does not work.

One night as we were preparing to go to bed, I had a knack for something sweet. I rooted around the pantry while she went to the master bathroom. I do not know how they got there, but as chance would have it there were some Oreo cookies in the jar. I grabbed a couple and put the lid back on. Clink. *Why don't they make rubber cookie jar lids?* I was sure I was busted, caught red-handed in the cookie jar like some preschooler. If she heard it, she never said anything. She did not need to. I was already deep in self-chatter by the time I stood before the bathroom mirror brushing my teeth. I had reached a new low: I was now sneaking food in my own home. *What have I become?* I vowed not to go down that road anymore. I would not hide my eating, pretending that I was somehow performing an act of kindness by not having it confront her. If I was eating a cookie, I was eating a cookie whether or not she saw me or cared. This parasitic disorder would not claim me host. I would eat, or not eat, by my own choice.

The second thing that was unveiling in me was that I do indeed enjoy the dining experience. This is not something that was uniquely my wife's domain. I own this too. I like having a family meal together at home. I value the traditional Thanksgiving. And I do enjoy dining out. Perhaps I enjoy dining out a little too much. That was a revelation gifted to me during these later stages of recovery. I do not particularly care all that much about the food itself, but I do like the restaurant experience. It does not need to be fancy. Pizza joints can be as welcome as the steak house. I simply enjoy spending time with my wife or family in a restaurant, where others have to busy themselves over the preparation and cleanup. There does not need to be deep conversation or swooning music. I just like to kick back a bit at the end of the day, or the end of the week, or just about any time. By comparison, if I have to eat alone in a restaurant while on business travel, it is a nightmare. I would almost rather select from the vending machines and retreat to my hotel room. This was all news to me. I had not given these things much thought before the surgery, and certainly had not expected to look at them later on. But they were surfacing despite my intentions, and I needed to be honest with myself and those around me. Although I would not live or die if I had to give up anything in particular, taken as a whole I had to admit that yes, I did have some food likes that I wanted to keep enjoying in the future, and yes, I did like dining out as a form of entertainment. I wanted to continue on with these things in some form in my future if that was at all possible.

The egg episode became larger than life for me. It marked there was a future where we could have real meals of reduced portions together. As the medical diet progressed on to more and more solid foods, I began to let go of the guilt I felt in eating full course meals with her smaller portions. Pork chops made it back on the menu. We could dine out. But most importantly, the egg signified a change in my own awareness. The old me that thought I did not care at all about food had died and new revelations were hatching. The symbolism was surreal.

LET'S (NOT) TALK ABOUT SEX

Wouldn't you prefer to floss your dog's teeth or do something else rather than read this section? Please? Well, if you have stuck with it this far, then I am obligated to share with you. I will do my best, but it will not be easy.

Let me begin by stating I was generally happy with our sex life at the time. All relationships have ebbs and flows, and about the only thing the "sexperts" seem to agree on is that everything varies according to the individual. Once you separate the fantasy from the reality, I had to admit that my sex life seemed pretty normal, and I had no reason to complain.

When we discussed the surgery together at the outset, one item that she identified as a possible benefit to weight loss was an enhanced energy level in the bedroom. That was interesting. I would not bet the ranch on it, but if it came about, I was not going to complain about it either. This was at least something pleasant to think about. So, like any guy, I would think about it often. If there is anything I have learned in life, it is that every coin has two sides, and you better look at them both. So of course, a new worry arose in me as I pondered the flip side. If there was this incredible weight loss, and this newly vitalized sexual energy, could it threaten the marriage? Would her coworkers make advances; moreover, would she resist? Could she embrace this newly found energy only with me? My mind began to wander in bad places, all living in a future that had not yet been born. Settle down, I told myself. I would go through this one day, and then onto the next.

The doctors said we could resume sexual relations whenever we felt comfortable. I hate it when they say that. I would have felt better if they said, "Refrain for 3 weeks minimum." At least then I would have felt like I was getting our money's worth. For us, I recall the right time was someplace between weeks four and five. It was a clumsy, hesitant affair on my part, and I was more nervous than on my wedding night. The surgical areas had healed well, but there were other complexities. I was self-conscious about any touching of the abdomen. Hips and legs were uncooperative and uncomfortable, so the entire game of positioning became a distraction. It would take some more time to get back to where we once were. Time marched onward.

I was a weight-loss idiot. It never occurred to me that when one experiences a rapid weight loss, they lose weight everywhere. When she or I gained weight, it seemed a gradual thing, and the changes were barely noticeable in our sexual relations. We adjusted as we went along, all without a fuss.

Now that weight loss was accelerating, there was a substantial change. Things changed almost weekly, and what was good last time did not seem pleasurable for her this time. Performance anxiety of a new sort was creeping in. I felt I was fumbling about miserably. I wondered if any other man had ever "lost his touch." I began to worry more about my shortcomings. Instead of a new sexual energy, what we were experiencing was a parallel escalation in our own individual performance anxieties.

We worked hard to keep lines of communication open. The injustices of middle age were creeping into our sex life, so we had a tangled web of weight-loss, middle-age, and insecurity issues to plow through. On one or two occasions we made deliberate decisions to take a break from sexual activity for a while, just to help sort things out. Those were good decisions, and we always came back together better for them.

FINDING THE GROOVE

The first year was coming to a close. She apparently knew how much she should eat of what, and had the skill set necessary for success. There were only three or four times that I could tell dinner did not set quite right. The first time caught me by surprise because of how quickly her discomfort set in, but after that I knew how it presented. I made conscious decisions <u>not</u> to look for signs of discomfort. It was not my business to monitor what or how she was eating.

We both have an affinity for a nicely chilled, iced 44-ounce cup of diet cola. It is one of our twin vices. This was one item I thought best to indulge at work rather than at home. One day, one of those 32-ounce soda cups from the convenience store followed her home. I challenged it, reminding how the doctor told us not to drink soda. We reached for the surgery information packet, and her point was affirmed. The concern was not really about the carbonation stretching out the stomach, but rather that primarily it was a poor food choice. It took up space could be better used by a protein snack. Sodas had caffeine, empty calories, blah blah blah. I thought there was a physical risk, but that seemed to be a minor point covered by some sentence like, "we don't have data regarding whether or not soda can lead to stretching of the stomach." So long as we were in the arena of food choices, it was not to be my business. At first, I was angry about it. How could you risk what you have worked for? In a short time, my anger and my self-righteousness would yield.

With more food choices possible, there also came dessert samplings, especially when dining out. On the occasions when our daughter was able to join us for a dinner out, we frequently had the dessert triad. In its dysfunction, it worked this way:

[Dad, breaking the ice] I think I'd like to have dessert tonight, if it doesn't bother you.

[Mom] Sure, no problem.

[Dad] I think I'd like to get my own piece, OK?

[Mom] Yeah, that's fine. Daughter-unit, do you want to share something?

[Daughter glances to Dad seeking non-verbal cues. Daughter stammers…] Uh, well, hmmm…

[Dad] Dearest wife, if you want something, I really, really do not mind paying full price for it even if you just want a bite or two. Honest.

[Mom] Oh I know, but I hate to waste a whole piece for just a bite. Daughter, were you thinking of anything?

[Daughter] Well, the carrot cake was looking rather good, I must say.

[Mom] Or how about the chocolate explosion? What would you think about sharing that?

[Waiter, interrupting] Have we reached any decisions here tonight?

[Dad] Yes. I will have the orange-key-lime thing.

[Waiter] And you ma'am?

[Mom] Nothing thanks. Just bring an extra spoon.

[Waiter] And you Miss?

[Daughter] I will pass, thanks.

[Dad to daughter] If **you** want to order something, then you should feel free to order it. Really!

[Daughter] No, no, it is ok. Thanks.

[Waiter, sensing angst, retreats quickly to the safety of the kitchen. Father fails to rescue daughter and falls on his sword. Daughter fails to order chocolate and decides to join a nunnery instead of talking to her mother. Mom does not really believe what just happened and seems angry, either at herself or at the family. The meal ends in tragedy.]

We tried to work through this, but in my view, we had mixed success. It was important to me to get our daughter out from the "sharing circle." I understood my wife would not be comfortable ordering her own dessert, not because of the cost or waste, but because she was not ready to have an entire dessert presented to her and take only a bite or two. The best possible compromise seemed to be for her and me to share, planning that as far ahead as possible in the meal.

A TAILORED LIFESTYLE

The active adult lifestyle bug has not bitten us yet. We are not living the life I had quite imagined, or that the doctors would probably have me live. I guess I have to do it my way after all. So far, I have lived rather successfully.

The kids are on their own, and we are relatively new empty nesters. Work occupies a substantial portion of our lives still. We have yet to join a hiking club or anything similar, so I personally faltered in my goal of becoming more active with my wife. She maintains an exercise routine, which I greatly admire. I hate indoor exercise.

The complexities of managing food, cooking and whatnot have been greatly simplified now that there are only two of us in the house. We both are eating smaller portions that are higher in protein. These are "real meals," and every sit-down dinner with my wife is a special time I do not take for granted. We enjoy dining out as it suits our whims.

I wish to declare ice cream to be a vegetable. Face the facts; everyone's life will be easier if I do. I like to have a sweet treat before bed, at 9:17 PM to be specific (which coincides with the second commercial break of whatever TV show we are watching at 9:00 PM). And a bowl of ice cream is a first-place winner. I am not sure if this is something I grew up with, something I brought into the relationship, or something that evolved later on, but make no mistake about it—this is a reliable pattern. Even the dog knows when it is 9:17, and she patiently awaits her treat at the same time.

We have danced around the 9:17 snack for years. Do I get up and get it, or will she? Do I get just my own? Do I ask? Do we put it on the shopping list, or just act surprised when it appears in the freezer? High fat or low fat? Syrup or not? Just once a week on Fridays? I wanted to challenge my enabling behavior, and so I stopped participating in the ritual for a time. Things did not appear to change on the other side of the street, and after a while I went back in.

Recently, we decided to try a one-month experiment without sugar. This was a good challenge for me, since I had never really tried something like this. Is this something like dieting? I noticed that my weight had settled on one of those set-points I preferred was lower, so now I would take the time to weigh in, something I had never done more than 10 times a year in my life. I began to check food labels for sugar content. The 9:17 snack was outlawed, of course. In short, I was trying to experience what some aspects of life might be like in her world. I made it through my 30 days, crowning my victory with a nice, sweet piece of cheesecake that probably had every calorie I had forestalled. Was it worth doing the experiment? Yes, it was. It was worth it because I took the chance to try experiencing it from someone else's perspective, a view that I can only approximate but never fully understand. It was worth it because I found my own temptations, and my own inner voices to deal with them. And it was worth it because the 9:17

PM snack surfaced again without me. Maybe it was not really all my fault after all.

Things are not quite as black and white as they once were. Dessert, in and of itself, is not the embodiment of evil. Soda does not apparently make people explode. I know I cannot control what my wife chooses to eat any more than I could force my children to eat vegetables.

I have come closer to understanding eating disorders and food obsession. Closer than ever before, and faster than the prior 20 years. I have looked into my wife's eyes and seen glimpses of her never-ending struggle. She never gets a break; her mind never rests. The monkey is relentlessly on her back. I get it now: it never lets up. I have great empathy for her, and for all afflicted.

I no longer live with the specter that whatever I do is the prevailing enabling behavior that will lead to her demise. I cannot save her. Truth be told, we have good days and bad days. Sometimes we have days with ice cream and pork chops, and sometimes it is just fish. But every day, we work together and push forward as best as we can. I try hard to be true to myself, keep my slate clean, and not to trip her up along her journey. This is a life we are both enjoying. Neither of us is quitting.

And I do pray that I am not deluding myself. For if I am wrong, and my sweet tooth winds up being the straw that breaks the camel's back, I greatly fear that final outcome.

EPILOGUE

This was going to be fairly easy writing, I told myself. And I was right—for only the first 500 words. In writing, I discovered I have a lot of energy tied up inside. Anger at this disease, or affliction, or disorder, or whatever it is. Anger at its causes, and its results. And a great sadness for anyone caught in its grips. Retelling my "pork chop episode" still makes my eyes well with tears for reasons I do not even want to try and understand, but I am sure that will be a journey for me.

Despite the struggles, the sadness, and the confusion, there is indeed happiness that rises above. This is a point I may have failed to emphasize properly. When I look today, we have come an exceptionally long way. We are healthier than we were years ago. Yes, we have our faults and may not be text-book recovery examples, but we are in recovery. And that is a beautiful thing: to be able to get better without needing to be perfect.

OTHER JOURNEYS

RENEE

I received training as a Bariatric RN but decided at 280# that all I needed to do was eat right, exercise and the weight would come off. I certainly did NOT need surgery to accomplish that! After 2 years AND losing/regaining the same 25 pounds in 3 separate attempts – I was hopeless and defeated. One day, I got on my beloved horse to take a ride. She staggered and groaned when I heaved myself into the saddle. I sat there and sobbed. I knew my denial had been broken for the last time. I WAS morbidly obese and could not lose weight and keep it off. I needed help!

I live in Colorado but chose to travel to the surgeon group in Florida that trained our Bariatric team. I knew that having surgery was a big step and needed to be performed by a skilled surgeon and support team. Traveling to a Center of Excellence Bariatric program was worth every penny that I spent.

My medical insurance company excluded WLS completely from the policy. I had to pay cash. The surgeon's office was really helpful with presenting different options to cover costs. I chose to get a home equity loan. In order to save my life, I needed surgery sooner rather than waiting until I could save that kind of cash on my own.

On Dec 6, 2006 I went into the operating room. Dr Marema performed a RNY Gastric Bypass. I was excited and determined to be a successful WLS patient. Everything went very well. Soon I was in my hospital room calling friends around the country to tell them "I DID IT!"

As a new WLS postop, I followed all the rules. I had done my research beforehand. I was ready to tackle morbid obesity and win! My actual experience turned out in line with what I expected. The weight began melting off my body. The overwhelming fatigue was difficult to cope with while working fulltime and living my life. This took months to resolve. Emotionally, I was happy/excited and enjoying every moment of my WLS honeymoon period. I made sure I ate a healthy low carb food plan recommended by my Bariatric surgeon. I did not touch anything with sugar listed as an ingredient. I also made sure to incorporate daily exercise to save what muscle mass I could and establish a strong habit.

Within the first year postop, I lost 125# and reached my goal weight of 150#. When my body released the physical insulation, my emotions became raw. My emotional struggles were intense and forced me to seek help from a counselor. Slowly, I began to discover the emotional reasons behind my obesity. This aspect of my life required healing as well. I had to be willing to enlist other sources for support. 12-step programs, a WLS Life Coach and expanding my spirituality are all part of my "team". I cannot do this alone. And my Higher Power does not require me to have all the answers.

This journey has not been all upward and forward. I relapsed back into depression and eating sugar. Yes, it made me sick, but the emotional pain needed soothing. I refused to just give up! I kept trying. I kept getting up each time I fell face down in a bowl of chocolate. I did not give in to the despair when I saw the weight coming back on my body for a total regain of #50. I grit my teeth and keep fighting even when I felt like a huge WLS failure.

This leads me to discuss what has not worked for me as a WLS postop. Reintroducing "healthy" whole grain carbohydrates? My body reacts strongly, and I dive into them quickly. And the healthy choices lead directly to unhealthy carbohydrate choices. As I become more enthralled to sugary foods, my body, mind, and spirit suffer. This is my experience.

Being completely "black and white" with my food and exercise plan does not work either. I am overly critical of myself. The slightest deviation will result in harsh judgment and self-talk. This attitude leads quickly to self-sabotage.

Gently allowing myself to unfold has been vital to my long-term recovery. Even though the ride gets rough at times, I have NEVER regretted my choice to have WLS. I have my life back and it is opening in miraculous ways!

I asked some people the following questions:

APRIL

What factors went into your decision to have bariatric surgery?

There were several factors that went into my decision to have gastric bypass surgery. One of them was my health, my blood pressure kept creeping higher and higher, border line diabetes, back and leg pain. I also went on a long weekend with my mom and sisters. Several pictures of us together, I was huge and embarrassed, but the major decision was my health. I wanted to be around for my family, especially my husband, children, and grandchildren.

When did you have your surgery (how long ago)?

I had my surgery on December 21, 2004.

Was the actual experience in line with what you expected? If not, how was it different?

Yes.

What changes have you successfully made in your lifestyle? (What is Working?)

My routine. I am very routine driven, as long as I stay on my routine I can stay on track with my eating, supplements, and exercise. I try to remember to ask myself if I am really hungry, what is going on at the time I want something to eat –

does not always work. Also, if there are trigger foods in the house, I put them in a place that is very inconvenient to get to, usually a place high in the pantry, where I have to get a chair and climb up to get to them. Stress has a huge impact on my life and how I deal with issues and food.

What changes have you tried but found them to be not helpful? (What's not Working?)

I have a real problem with journaling and keeping track of my food, supplements, water, and exercise. I will do well for a couple days but cannot seem to make it any further than that.

Knowing what you know now, would you do it again?

YES, in a heartbeat!

CATHERINE

What factors went into your decision to have bariatric surgery?

I felt captive in my own body. My life had become "smaller" as I was unwilling to participate in my own life to the degree I wished to. I was about to have more grandchildren and I wanted to be an active participant in their lives, not limited by my weight. I also wanted to no longer be embarrassed by my size. To feel comfortable being me.

When did you have your surgery (how long ago)?

July 2008

Was the actual experience in line with what you expected? If not, how was it different?

Yes, I did experience a slower recovery due to a diagnosis of pericarditis, which was unrelated to the surgery.

What changes have you successfully made in your lifestyle? (What is Working?)

EXERCISE! After the first 40 or so pounds lost, I started working out in the pool, then started walking, then cycling. I am enjoying exercise for the first time in my life! This is definitely working. It helps with weight control, and appetite control and gives me a better sense of overall wellbeing.

Knowing what you know now, would you do it again?

YES, absolutely!

Is there anything important about your experience that these questions have not addressed?

Weight re-gain is a constant battle, made much harder if I am not vigilant about the exercise component. At about 2 years out, I stopped being as careful with the "rules" (i.e., eat protein first, no sugar, and no snacks). That is exactly when the re-gain began. Still fighting the constant need to eat.

SANDY

What factors went into your decision to have bariatric surgery?

It is kind of a funny story because I had never really thought about it, until a friend started thinking and talking about it. It was her interest that elicited my desire for the surgery. Interestingly enough, she did not have the surgery right away. She thought she would give it one more try before having the surgery. So, she went to a weight loss program and lost a bunch of weight. I, in the meantime, had totally given up on diets and could get to feeling really hopeless sometimes. My friend did end up having the surgery, but not until about two years after I did.

When did you have your surgery (how long ago)?

February 13, 2008 (Note...there is no chocolate in the hospital, even on Valentine's Day!)

Was the actual experience in line with what you expected? If not, how was it different?

I remember being curious about some things like, would I still burp? Could I manage the pain medications? How long would I be off work? When could I eat again? Yes, I still burped. As I recall, I did not need the pain medication more than just a few days after I got home. I was in the hospital two nights and on a morphine pump (self-administered) which helped a lot with the pain in the hospital. I went back to work after about three weeks. So, physically, the experience was in line with what I expected. The emotional recovery was another matter entirely. I do not think anyone can prepare you for what the experience will be like. I had given up my best friend, in the interest of better health and living longer.

What changes have you successfully made in your lifestyle? (What is Working?)

I worked with a nutritionist for a while. That helped get me in touch with the rebel in me that just wanted to eat, eat, eat! We worked with portion control and food choices. My plan with her contained LOTS of protein, which seemed to help a bit with my sugar cravings. Exercise is an important part of my recovery, even though I am good at talking myself out of doing it from time to time. I have significantly widened my support system, talking with other women who have had weight-loss surgery. There are listservs available and groups online that I became a part of. Therapy helps a LOT.

What changes have you tried but found them to be not helpful? (What's not Working?)

Trying to monitor what I eat every day; all day long makes me crazy. 12-Step groups were not helpful for me, though they are great for some people. Trying to hide from my problems and feelings is not working. When I have uncomfortable emotions, I still want to overeat. Grazing (eating small portions but eating all day long) can still put the weight on, so I have to be really careful.

Knowing what you know now, would you do it again?

At first, I was not really sure since the emotional adjustment has been so difficult. But then I remember how much it improved my health, and I say "of course!"

Is there anything important about your experience that these questions have not addressed?

I do not mean to sound grim or discouraging in talking about the emotional adjustment I had to make. It is all a part of the process. I was overeating to stuff down my feelings. Of course, I am not going to want them to surface to the light of day. But slowly and surely, I am meeting some of my emotions, often for the first time, and understanding that the pain is not in the feeling. The pain is in the resistance to the feeling. And one piece of advice to those who are getting ready to have their surgery: be careful about "The Last Supper" mindset. I went to ALL my favorite restaurants before I had my surgery, since I knew it would be a long time before I frequented them again, if ever! I gained several pounds right before surgery due to "The Last Supper" syndrome.

KASSANDRA

What factors went into your decision to have weight-loss surgery?

I had tried everything that I knew of, with no success. Any weight I lost came back, almost immediately. I was physically fatigued at all times, and very depressed. I did not see a huge risk, but I did not mind if there was. I honestly did not care if I died in surgery...as long as I did not have to live like that anymore.

When did you have your surgery?

Eight years ago, September 9, 2003.

Was the actual experience in line with what you expected?

The experience of surgery and losing weight was pretty much in line with what I had heard, except for some unexpected back pain a few days after surgery that lasted only about two days. I do not think I had spoken with anyone who was more than two years out, so I did not expect my appetite would come back the way it did. About five years after surgery, I started gaining weight. I was unemployed, which I am sure contributed, and I found myself eating almost constantly and could not stop. I found myself 18 pounds over my goal weight, which I had achieved and maintained for some time.

What changes have you successfully made in your lifestyle? (What is Working?)

I have reactive hypoglycemia, so I have found that restricting carbohydrates and eliminating all sugars are necessary for my health and well-being. Eating this way also helps maintain my weight loss. I wear a Fitbit pedometer at all times and find the data tracking tools on their website invaluable. I have taken a job that keeps me active, so I walk 9-10,000 steps/day and eat ~1200 calories/day, which I find fairly comfortable (thanks to *my smaller stomach). I do *not* restrict fat at all, just carbohydrates and total calories, and following this lifestyle, I have successfully lost 14.5 pounds in the last few months. 3.5 pounds to goal!*

What changes have you tried but found them to be not helpful? (What's not Working?)

Trying to become someone I am not. I have tried to become a "fitness buff"/" gym rat", but I cannot stick to it, because I do not enjoy it. I find exercise boring, and I do not like to sweat. The pedometer method works for me, and sometimes I meet my goal without trying. If not, I walk inside my house, in air-conditioned comfort, without the added effort of changing clothes or going anywhere, and I do not have to pay for a gym membership.

Knowing what you know now, would you do it again?

In a heartbeat!

Is there anything important about your experience that these questions have not addressed?

Surgery is not a magic pill and does not resolve any psychological food issues one may have. While it physically prevents you from overeating for a time, eventually you will be able to overeat and regain weight. I thought I would never have to count calories again, but I was wrong...even so, it is much easier to maintain a healthy weight (and a healthy eating plan) than it ever was before.

RECOVERY – WHAT'S NOT WORKING

There are several things I tried on my weight-loss surgery journey, both pre- and post-surgery. As noted, I have dealt with my eating disorder for a long time. Despite my countless efforts to rid myself of its power, it has persisted. Whatever "caused" it, wherever it came from, it has at times been very much in my foreground and other times more in the background. Some of the following examples you might need to try out for yourself, but if you can learn from my mistakes and not make them yourself, all the better. So, on to a discussion of what was not helpful.

THE LATEST DIET

When I was doing research on the different bariatric procedures and trying to decide which procedure I wanted, I remember reading about this food plan where you could shrink your stomach pouch after stretching it out from eating too much. This was for people, I believe, who had had the lap-band surgery or the gastric bypass, both of which work by creating a small pouch at the top of your stomach for food. This plan was a way to get back to basics with your eating and get back on track after some straying. It essentially replicates your first few weeks after surgery in five days, consuming only liquids the first two days, then soft proteins on day three, firm proteins on day four and hard proteins on day five. I decided against those two types of weight-loss surgery because I was not going to be a person who had to worry about dieting after my surgery (so I thought). The vertical sleeve gastrectomy created a cylinder out of your stomach instead of a pouch and was not supposed to stretch out. That was the procedure I wanted. I really believed that I was going to be through with that diet mentality. This could not be further from the truth. I am certainly trying to be rid of the diet mentality, but that is because it does not work, not because I am satisfied with my weight.

The other reason I wanted to have the sleeve surgery is that, since there was no rerouting of the intestines, one would not experience "dumping syndrome." This is something that happens in many gastric bypass patients. When a lot of sugar is consumed the pancreas produces insulin rapidly and this insulin dumps into the bloodstream much quicker that it normally would. Dumping syndrome is characterized by flu-ish type symptoms and, from what I gather, is not fun. The doctors who do not understand eating disorders, thinks that this acts as a deterrent to eating too much sugar, and for some people it likely does. What I was afraid of was that I would want sugar badly enough that I would eat it, anyway, fully knowing the consequences.

As I have said, I lost 80 pounds in the first nine months after my surgery. I have a lot of euphoric recall about those nine months, because from this perspective now they seem like they were blissful. I often long for those days again when life seemed so simple. There were not food decisions to make. I just had to drink that disgustingly sweet, syrupy liquid form of protein, a few times a day for the first two weeks. Then, remember, I got to add one egg to my day for week three. I actually dropped 30 pounds in the first three weeks, which I do not believe is typical. They call this the "honeymoon period" and it is aptly named. Yet, this period of time only qualifies as a honeymoon period in hindsight. As I think honestly about it now, when I was going through it, I was not all that blissful.

My first problem during this "honeymoon period," as I have said, was that I was hungry, and they had promised me I would not be. With the hormone ghrelin gone there would be no appetite. People I knew who had had surgery were talking about not being hungry. My surgery buddy, who I met in the hospital, was not hungry. The people coming to the surgery support group were not hungry. Why was I the only one who was hungry? It was not even the hunger that was so much the problem, as it was that I was so mad about it. My eating disorder believed that the only way to survive eating bird-size portions of food was to not be hungry. I felt cheated, and I was mad. Once I had graduated from the protein syrup to regular protein shakes, I tried a lot of things to help with the hunger. I tried putting a tablespoon of peanut butter or half a banana in the shake. I tried drinking my breakfast later in the morning. I tried small snacks in between the protein shakes. All of these things helped but did not explain why I was hungry to begin with. My eating disorder knew why I was hungry. It was because I was STARVING myself to death! I had just had 85% of my stomach physically removed from my body! FOREVER! What was I thinking??? It is recommended that one not ask a person who has had weight-loss surgery if they are glad about it until they are past the six-month mark. That would certainly hold true for me.

So, I was hungry, against all physiological probabilities. Second, my eating disorder was complaining nonstop about how much food I could not eat. It took about six months for my stomach and my eating disorder to come to a compromise. At six months, I could finally eat a bit more and be satisfied with a bit less. I knew more about what I could hold so I would take more reasonable portions and not have to leave a lot of food on my plate. I would get my takeout box in the restaurant at the beginning of my meal instead of at the end. That way I could pack up what I was not going to eat right away and not have it mocking me on my plate later.

Eight months after my surgery, with 20 pounds still that I wanted to lose, my weight lost stopped. I was not happy. I wanted to know why it had stopped. What was I doing wrong? How could I fix it? I postulated all sorts of explanations. Maybe it was because all of those "good" habits I had acquired after the surgery (no caffeine, no diet soda, and very little sugar, less restaurant eating) had begun to slip and the "bad" habits started to creep back in. Maybe it was because I could eat larger portions now and things were leveling off. Maybe the "set point" theory was right, and this was what my body *wanted* to weigh. Maybe it was because Mercury was in retrograde. (I am not an astrological person myself, but people tell me that bad things happen when Mercury is in retrograde!) There had to be a reason that my weight loss stopped, but even more important was trying to figure out how to get it started again.

That is when the diet mentality started to creep back in. I tried that "back to basics" food plan I had read about, despite my original belief that I would never have to do that. I tried it a few times over the next several months. The first time I tried it, I was able to do all five days. I even lost a few pounds, though it clearly states that the intention is not to lose weight but to get the feel of your pouch back and help it work as a tool again. The next few times I tried it I found it exceedingly difficult to get through the first two days of only liquids. I was plenty used to solid food at every meal by now and was not interested in giving that up, even for just a mere few days. So, that was not working.

My weight stabilized for about a year. I seemed to have a few pounds that I would gain and lose, but that was probably more a function of how often I weighed myself. Then, in October 2009, 20 months after my surgery, the Halloween candy hit the stores and I was a goner. My eating disorder decided that I was entitled to eat Halloween candy and I bought some early in October. Well, that candy never saw Halloween. I had to buy more for the trick-or-treaters, but there were not a lot of them, so I had candy left over and ate that as well. A funny side story is that even before my surgery I was thinking about the size of the pouch that I would be left with and figured that the pouch would be big enough to hold a miniature Milky Way! So that October began a long, slow weight gain that amounted to about 12 pounds by the time another year had gone by. I am convinced that the reason I had not gained more weight than that is that my eating disorder was still strong enough to keep my eating "in control" at least some of the time.

As my weight began to increase, I desperately wanted to find the magic diet. My diet mentality was alive and well. I decided a few times to go back to the popular weight loss program I had been to before, but I never did. I decided a few times to give up sugar, but I never did that either. I was on the lookout for the perfect diet and scoured magazines and the internet. Recently, I heard about some people who were losing a lot of weight on the latest and greatest diet. The weight loss claims were "lose 30 pounds in 30 days." I wanted to lose 30 pounds (the 20 I never lost plus the 10 I put back on), so this was very tempting. It seemed, though, like such a drastic, restrictive plan that I reluctantly talked myself out of it. My eating disorder never really wanted me to diet; it just wanted me to lose weight. There had to be a way to do that without having to give up the things I still wanted to eat! There was not. Looking for the next, latest, and greatest diet was not working.

"FROM NOW ON AND FOREVER…"

Going right along with the latest and greatest diet for me is the idea of "From now on, and forever…" Whenever I think, however innocently, "I'll just do this with my food…," my brain automatically adds "…FOREVER." I am left, then, with a standard I cannot possibly live up to. I cannot maintain any behavior forever. No one can. I am destined to fail, by the very design of that assumption, and fail I do, over and over again.

In my dieting days, as I mentioned, I would use a blank food journal to write down what I ate. Every week when I went to the meeting, I would get a brand new, BLANK journal. I got to start all over again and try to be "perfect" for another week. The imperfections of the previous week no longer mattered. They had been tucked away, shelved. No one would see them, and I did not have to talk about them. I could just start over and renew my battle cry of "From now on and forever...." And every week I had more things to do "from now on and forever." From now on and forever I would do the program perfectly. From now on and forever I would weigh and measure everything. From now on and forever I would eat perfectly, exercise perfectly, even drink water perfectly! Then, when I was not able to do all this perfectly, I thought I was "bad" and shame ("I'm broken.") plagued me. This shame and need to be perfect was about more than just food, as I will elaborate on in a little bit. The food, however, was where it manifested itself the strongest and the longest.

PICK YOUR FAVORITE SYMPTOM

Compulsive overeating. If looking for the latest and greatest diet was not working, perhaps the answer was to not restrict what I was eating at all. If I felt horribly deprived and subsequently rebelled at the mere *thought* of a diet, my eating disorder logic told me, then *not* trying to control what I ate seemed to be the next thing to try. The problem with that was that I gravitated toward so much sugar when I tried this that the weight continued to reappear. I did have some times of paying attention to getting fruit and vegetable servings and figuring out how much protein I was eating. These were times when I felt good about how I was eating and felt good about myself. Always in the background, though, was eating disorder noise about my sugar intake, and my weight was slowly increasing despite my efforts to eat reasonably. I felt entitled to eat what I wanted. I was an adult. I had lived a life of dieting and being overweight. I had had surgery and lost a ton of weight. This entitlement, though, fueled overeating. I would eat what I wanted, when I wanted it, and consequences be damned! I wanted to ignore the consequences, but I could not. Regaining weight was not acceptable on any level, to me or to my eating disorder. My eating disorder wanted to ply me with all the shame messages that came with overeating. "You're weak." "You're bad." "You'll never lose weight again." "You're going to gain it all back, you just wait." To my *non*-eating disorder self, regaining the weight simply was not ok. I really wanted to be able to pay attention to what I ate, without being obsessed. I wanted to maintain the health benefits I had achieved. I wanted to feel good about myself and how I looked. I *did* feel that way sometimes. I liked it. I wanted to feel it more.

Compulsive exercise. My eating disorder wished I could become a compulsive exerciser. I had met some compulsive exercisers. Physically, they looked fairly good to me. This was about the magical belief that if I just exercised *enough*, the weight would fall off and I could continue to eat anything I wanted. My eating disorder was always trying to maneuver a way for me to eat as much as I wanted and not be overweight. Would exercise do it? There was one period of time before my surgery where I walked on the treadmill 30 minutes a day, six days a week (which was as compulsive as I could get). I only lost about two pounds in over six weeks. That was not nearly enough to make it worth all that effort.

After surgery I tried again. I exercised as often as I could make myself, which usually amounted to 3-4 times per week (hardly what anyone could call compulsive, but I still wanted to be!). I rode the stationary, recumbent bicycle so I could read at the same time. I treasured this reading time. I would read mysteries, and when I was on the bike was the only time I would let myself read. So, I would exercise, but the fact that my legs were moving was inconsequential. I did it only so I could read.

I also lifted small weights and did a routine that a trainer had worked with me on. Personal training was helpful and gave me some guidelines to follow. My motivation, however, waxed, and waned and some days it was all I could do to force myself to work out. The quality of the book I was reading was often the deciding factor if I would exercise or not. I joined a health club and would often go there after work. I even carpooled with a coworker and we met in the morning at the club, one of us drove us to work from there, and we ended up back at the club after work. This made it much easier to exercise, yet still I was on again, off again. I would never make a good compulsive exerciser. I could not even make a good regular exerciser.

Restricting. My eating disorder also wanted me to be anorexic. Now, I fully understand that anorexics have their own form of hell that they go through every day, but my eating disorder does not know that. My eating disorder told me that if I could just stop eating, life would be so much simpler. It would be blissful to never *want* to eat. Not eating at all seemed like it would be so much easier than having to make all these good choices all the time, day in and day out, week after week, year after year. Being healthy is exhausting if you have an eating disorder. There had to be a time of relief from the effort. People talked about "eating to live" rather than "living to eat." That is what I wanted. I just had no idea how to do that.

My "restricting" was always part of the eating disorder cycle. I would overeat, feel guilt and shame, decide I had to do better and then try to restrict what I was eating. I would skip a meal. I would eat the dessert and not the main course. I often wondered if I dispensed with the healthy food altogether and just ate chocolate, maybe then I would not gain weight. Calories in, calories out. If you take in fewer calories than you expend you will lose weight, and vice versa. I was not a particularly good restrictor, because I was a compulsive overeater at heart. What felt like restricting to me probably looked like normal eating to someone without an eating disorder. I had no concept of reality when it came to food. Was I really "binging" when I ate one candy bar? Was I really "restricting" when I waited until 9am to eat a snack, having skipped breakfast at 630am? Certainly, I could not physically binge in the literal definition of the term. I could not consume a lot of food at one time, but I could sure feel out of control with what I *was* eating. The weight was coming back. I was convinced that I was gaining weight every minute of every day. I could not eat in peace. I chastised myself for eating things I did not think I "should" eat, and I berated myself for not being able to restrict enough to lose the weight that I was gaining. All that shame fueled the fire for more overeating. It was an endless cycle. I coined the term the "emotional trifecta" to describe the anger, shame and fear I would constantly feel about my eating. Anger at the universe for my having an eating disorder. Shame at not being able to "just control it." And fear that I would NEVER get any better. Was I was destined to live in this cycle of overeating, anger, shame and fear, then more overeating FOREVER? And there were times, in my desperation that forever was not going to be for much longer. My eating disorder brought me to suicidal thinking numerous times. I made a decision that I was not going to live the rest of my life with an active eating disorder. Without the tools, though, to arrest the disorder, the alternative was simply to not live longer.

Bulimia. As I mentioned, there was a period of time when I would make myself throw up, mostly in response to extreme physical discomfort. It was difficult for me initially to adjust to how little food I could eat, and I kept trying to eat more. It seemed that the line between enough food and too much was very thin indeed, sometimes only one bite different. There were times then when I would get overfull, extremely uncomfortable, and have to throw up. My eating disorder had secretly always wanted me to be bulimic, and it believed I had finally succeeded. I could overeat something I wanted, knowing I could get rid of it right afterwards. This seemed like the perfect solution to wanting to eat sugar and not wanting to be responsible for the consequences. This, however, did not prevent the weight gain that I was struggling with. Over time my stomach seemed to adjust quite readily to more food, so I very rarely needed to throw up anymore. I was not getting that overfull feeling, even after eating much more than I thought I should be able to. The truth is that eventually I could eat a small "normal" serving of just about anything. I no longer could consider myself restricted in the quantity of food I could eat. My perspective adjusted to understand that I could eat like a "normal" person (that is, a person who is NOT a compulsive overeater). I could not eat like I once did. I could not eat four pieces of pizza, but I could eat two, and that is twice what I thought I should be able to eat. I had to change how I was thinking about my eating. Before surgery, I assumed that I would always be restricted in the quantity of food that I could eat. I believed that my stomach was going to be in control of how much I ate. Perhaps that is why I thought I would not have to diet or watch what I ate. I was not going to have to control my food quantity. My stomach was going to do that for me. What became clear is that I *could* eat enough to regain weight. Whether it was because I was eating more in one portion or because I was eating more often during the day, my weight was slowly increasing. I had to pay attention. I had to be the one in control. My stomach was not going to control things for me.

TRANSFER ADDICTIONS

I have talked about my alcoholism. If I were still a drinker, it would have been quite easy to slip into problems with alcohol after my weight-loss surgery. Many people develop a transfer or a cross addiction once they have had bariatric surgery. Whether it is alcohol, other drugs, shopping, gambling, or compulsive sexual behaviors, people still seek an escape from the stresses of everyday life. The problem becomes that the addiction provides a stress of its own, and eventually the pursuit of that addiction takes over a person's life. People turn to addictive substances and behaviors in order to deal with stress, feelings, situations, relationships. The person gradually becomes so compelled by the addiction that any previously perceived benefit is far overshadowed by the discomfort the behavior brings. Once seen as a harmless "friend" the behavior has turned and become a foe. What initially seemed to help, then became a necessity, and eventually became a driven compulsion. The earmark of a strong addiction is that it keeps you alive, long enough to kill you.

I did not struggle with a transfer addiction per se, but I also did not gain any relief from my eating disorder. Sure, in the beginning I could not eat as much as I wanted, but food still consumed my thoughts and my feelings. Shame and perfectionism became complete obsessions, haunting me night and day. As my diet mentality returned, I thought incessantly about losing weight, either the weight that I had not lost yet, or the weight that was inching back on. Practically every bite I put in my mouth was placed on the "success" or "failure" side of my mental tabulator. And worrying about this day and night did a nice job of keeping me away from those feelings I did not want to feel. It worked like a smokescreen so I could not see what was really there.

RELYING ON MY INNER 5-YEAR-OLD

Sometimes I think all my food decisions were made by my "inner child." You have heard from her as you have been reading. Anytime I say "I want what I want when I want it" that is her. She likes cookies and candy and would have eaten them all day long if I had let her. She was on the side of my eating disorder that overate and made poor food choices. I mean, what did I expect? She is only five! Put a five-year-old, especially a sad one, in an adult body, with adult resources and adult money and you get a compulsive overeater. Pair her with the entitled attitude of "I earned this, and I deserve it" and you have got weight gain just waiting to happen.

She was sad still from childhood events and issues and, as I have discussed, food was an important focus in my life from an early age. I learned well the psychological benefits of overeating – comfort, solace, companionship. Food was social. It was nurturing. It bonded my family together when emotional difficulties were breaking us apart.

As I grew older, I began experimenting with drugs and alcohol and my eating disorder took a back seat for a while. Drugs and alcohol provided a much more pronounced escape from the stressors of my current life as well as from the ghosts of my past. Depending on a regular escape, though, eventually spiraled my life out of control, and I needed to get and stay clean and sober. When I did that, food was right there waiting for me to pick it up again.

Through this time, I was in and out of therapy, and I was meeting that sad inner five-year-old. I was getting the chance to heal from those childhood hurts. That took a long time and, in the meantime, that five-year-old wanted a lot of comfort, solace and companionship. We ate a lot of cookies and candy together, and my weight was always an issue.

Not only did it not work to let my inner-5-yr-old make my food decisions, but it was also not such a great idea for me to let her make other important decisions in my life either. She had the perspective and the coping skills of a five-year-old, and we did not fare very well when she was at the helm. She popped up when she got scared and tried to take over. She thought she knew what was best, but her judgment was limited by her age. When she was scared, she needed comfort and reassurance, yet not in the form of food as she thought. I could provide her what she needed if I listened to *me*, instead of letting her take control. As I listened to her fears and frights, I could calm and soothe her. How long had I used food to do just that! I needed to learn other ways to provide that comfort to her, and to myself.

WATCHING THE SCALE

Weighing myself made me crazy. Case in point: I had been working with a nutritionist and got weighed there once every two weeks. I saw this as my "official" weight, as I assumed her scale was more accurate than mine and the timing was consistent. Nevertheless, I weighed myself at home often and that was always first thing in the morning, without clothing and before coffee! Over the course of a couple of weeks, I had been really trying to rein myself in as far as sugar was concerned, and I had increased my exercise. I expected stellar results. At home, on a Wednesday when I weighed myself, I had lost 2.5 pounds! I was thrilled. Then, when I went to my nutritionist on Friday, my weight was back up and was exactly what I had weighed there two weeks earlier. That there can be up to a five-pound difference in my weight during the week, that seemingly has nothing to do with ANYTHING seems so unfair. Even if I had not weighed myself Wednesday, I would have been angry and frustrated that my weight had not changed after all the hard work I had done watching my sugar and increasing my exercise. I cannot tell if weighing myself Wednesday made it better, or worse, but either way I was not happy.

I had been known to weigh myself more than once a day, though that did not happen often. At home, I knew better than to weigh myself with clothes on, or when I had to go to the bathroom, or even just during the day rather than first thing in the morning. When I did have to weigh with clothes on, the clothes were carefully selected to be as lightweight as possible. No boots, no belts, no heavy jewelry. Then there were all the preparations for weighing. Drinking all the water I could possibly hold for days ahead of time, to flush any excess fluid out of my system. Then, not drinking any liquid at all within four hours of being weighed. I always wished I had been able to refrain from weighing more than once a week, but I did not find the willingness to do that. I had, at times, moved my scale out of my bathroom to a shelf in the closet, but it did not stay there. I had heard of some people, in recovery from their eating disorder, that were able to get rid of their scale altogether. That thought terrified me.

That magic number, though, could make or break my whole day. If the number was down, all was well with the world. If the number was up and sometimes even if it was just the same, then I was "bad" because I was not losing weight. I lived in fear of regaining ALL the weight that I lost. The minute I stopped losing weight, I became afraid of gaining it back. I do not think I had even *one minute* of rest at my lowest weight before that fear kicked in.

PERFECTIONISM

Somewhere in life I developed the belief that I needed to be perfect. If I were not perfect, I thought, people would not love me. If I were not perfect, people would go away, and I would be alone. Intellectually, of course, I knew I could not *be* perfect, so I mastered an elaborate defense that I thought allowed me to *seem* perfect. I worked many long, hard years in therapy to address the shame and the pain that came along with my being imperfect. The one place it still persisted, however, was with my eating disorder. This was shame's last stronghold. When I dieted, I had to do it perfectly or it was not worth doing. I had to exercise the perfect amount. I had to weigh myself the perfect number of times. I had to abstain from sugar perfectly. My weight had to be the perfect number. My body size and shape had to be perfect. All of this was in black and white, good, and bad, right, and wrong. There was no gray. There was no room for imperfection, for patient improvement, for baby steps. My eating disorder told me "It's my way, or the highway!" When all these things were not perfect, as I knew they simply could not be, then I was overcome with shame. My eating disorder would tell my inner five-year-old that she was "bad" and "wrong" and would not be loved. The eating disorder voice was merciless. Some people call it "the judge" or the "inner critic." Whatever metaphor works for you, this shaming, and critical voice tried to keep me in line by threatening me about people not loving me if I was not perfect. This inner voice believed that it *protected* me from being abandoned by making me behave perfectly.

SHAME AND SECRETS

So, the fact that I am not perfect *is a secret!* (You will not tell anyone, will you?) Keeping secrets kept me in shame. It kept me striving for that perfection and never reaching it. There is a familiar expression that "we are as sick as our secrets." Keeping something about me, or my behavior, secret came from a place of shame and also perpetuated it. How often I weighed myself was a secret because I felt shame about not doing it perfectly. Wearing clothes that did not fit kept me in shame. Clothes that were too big hid my imperfections that I felt shame about. Clothes that were tight reminded me that I had always struggled with my weight. I am sure you have heard people suggest using positive affirmations as a way to enhance self-esteem. Well, my eating disorder had perfected *negative* affirmations. "I am a weak and inferior person in the universe. I do not deserve to be loved or accepted the way I am. I am a hopeless, helpless individual with unlovable faults and imperfections." You get the idea. And my shame believed that those statements were FACTS. Shame did that. It told me things about myself that were not true but convinced me that they were. Shame protected me because if I believed those terrible things about myself, I would not venture out into the world, and if I did not venture out, I could not be abandoned. In some twisted way, my shame was designed to help keep me safe.

But it also factored into my overeating. I remember a time, early in my adult life, when I consciously understood that yelling at myself was the consequence for how I was eating. Almost like it was intentional, this yelling. I felt like I was eating "wrong" and yet I must not have been gaining weight at that time. So, the only negative consequence for my eating was my internal yelling. And I believed that there had to be a negative consequence. There had to be some "punishment" for how I was eating. Since the situation was not punishing me, by weight gain, then I would punish myself. Enter one of the vicious cycles of the eating disorder – that internal yelling came from a place of shame and those feelings of shame were so horrible and overwhelming that eating made them bearable. The shame caused me to overeat, which caused me more shame. The more I ate, the worse I felt, the more I ate. The overeating also dealt with the loneliness I felt in not being connected to people because I was afraid they would abandon me. Food was my friend. It was there for me 24 hours a day, 7 days a week, and 52 weeks a year. It never needed a vacation and it never let me down. I could turn to food in my darkest moments, and there were plenty of those with all the shame I felt about my overeating! No matter what I tried, I just could not seem to break that cycle. I worked with positive affirmations for a while and they really helped my self-esteem, but that did not spell my eating disorder. All the trauma work I did in therapy did not spell my eating disorder. The weight-loss surgery did not spell my eating disorder. My therapist and I believed that when I felt better about myself I would not "need" to overeat so much. But overeat I did, no matter how I felt. Food was celebration as well as solace. I could overeat for any reason, or for no reason at all! Why could I not control what I was eating? What was wrong with me? Was I so defective that I would never be well? It certainly seemed like it at times, and that was shame talking. Certainly, there was something "wrong" with me – I had an eating disorder! But shame took that a step further and told me that *I* was "bad" and "wrong" because I had an eating disorder. Shame convinced me that it was my "bad" behavior around food that *caused* my eating disorder. That, however, was not the case.

The causes for my eating disorder are numerous and varied and have to do with both genetics and environment. What the shame did was perpetuate my eating disorder. As I traveled on this recovery journey, I learned that there were things I could do to make my eating disorder better and there were things I could do to make it worse. I became quite accomplished at making it worse. I needed to focus next on what would make it better. Not *gone,* but better.

BLACK AND WHITE THINKING

In my eating disorder, the entire world was black or white. There was no gray. Food was either good or it was bad. I was either good or I was bad. I was either all the way on a diet, or all the way off. There was nothing in the middle. This food plan was either right or it was wrong. There was never doing only part of something. I either did it all or did nothing. Everything about me was "always" or "never." I would *always* be out of control with my eating. I would *never* find peace or serenity.

My alcohol and drug recovery reinforced this black and white thinking, because with alcohol and drugs it was either yes or no. There was no middle ground. I could not drink just a little. I had proved that countless times. I either drank way over the top, or I did not drink at all. In order to be sober, I had to abstain from alcohol and drugs completely.

Food was always (there is that word again!) different. I could not stop eating to gain control over my eating disorder, though

I certainly thought it would be easier if I could! They say with alcohol or drugs you can put the tiger in the cage, lock it up and throw away the key. With food, you have to take that tiger for a walk around the block three times a day. You could not do all-or-nothing with food. There had to be moderation, a middle ground, a hopefully peaceful coexistence.

There were certain foods that seemed to activate the eating disorder more than others, sugar being the primary item in that category. Even sugar, though, could not be all or nothing. Some people, I know, give up sugar entirely for a time, though I have not met anyone who could give it up forever. I was not willing to do that. Partly, it was an exceedingly difficult venture in our society. But I also genuinely believed that it was not about what I was putting in my mouth, but *why* I was overeating, that was the problem. Food, or more specifically – overeating – was meeting very concrete needs. I needed to meet those needs in other ways if I were to give up using food to meet them. First, I had to know what those needs were.

Food soothed what seemed to be a global anxiety that I felt. Perhaps as a result of earlier difficulties, my body seemed to be in a perpetual state of activation. There was an anxiety that agitated everything. After my depression was under control this anxiety surfaced, though it was not until several years later that I identified it as such. Food helped me deal with this anxiety. Food became how I took on the world. I could deal with any situation as long as I could overeat. The problem became that my eating disorder created MORE anxiety that I had to eat to soothe. Every time I was going to try another diet or food plan, I would become so anxious about failing yet again, that I overate. That accomplished two things. First, it soothed the anxiety about being afraid to fail. Second, it assured that failure, so I did not have to try! My eating disorder won. It maintained control. By creating so much anxiety about restricting my eating that I ended up overeating, my eating disorder made sure that I never tried to really follow anything that would provide any structure. Eating whatever I wanted whenever I wanted it was imperative, according to my eating disorder. I was able, at times, to follow a food plan for a few days, but not for longer than that. My eating disorder had a real dilemma though, because at the same time it wanted me to eat everything I wanted, it also wanted me to be thin. Time and time again, I proved that I could not do both. My eating disorder kept me trying, though. It kept convincing me that "this time it will be different." This time I will be able to follow the food plan and lose weight. But remember "from now on and forever"? When I added that phrase to "this time it will be different" I was off to the races again. And when I was not able to follow that plan from now on and forever, or for even more than just a few days, I would begin to overeat again, eating all that food that I had missed for that few days that I was on the plan.

SEARCHING FOR *THE* ANSWER

I kept thinking there was going to be ONE answer to my eating disorder. ONE reason, ONE cause, ONE solution. I kept looking for that answer. Every time I reached a new layer of insight in my therapy I thought "Surely, now I know what was driving my eating disorder, and now it will stop." It did not. Was the reason trauma? No. Was the reason addiction? No. Was the reason codependency? No. Was the reason shame? No. The reason, in fact, was *all* of those things. My eating disorder was fueled by sadness about my past, being uncomfortable and anxious in my present and worrying about my future. Since there was no one place to look for the cause, there was not going to be only one solution either. I was not going to stop therapy. I was not going to stop looking at and for contributing factors, but I had to give up the idea that I would find eternal peace right around the next corner, that *this* issue was finally the answer. I kept peeling the onion and going through layer after layer of the complexity of the human personality, only to discover more layers underneath. There was a core, a center that I had accessed from time to time. That core held the belief that "I do not matter." Changing that core belief would be a long, hard struggle, and would involve many layers of its own.

As I have talked about, I certainly thought that the weight-loss surgery was going to be THE answer. I believed that after the surgery, I would never have to diet or worry about what I ate again. I was going to BE thin, and I was going to STAY thin, with no effort or struggle. Nothing could be further from the truth. I find myself wondering now about whether I would have had the surgery if I had known it would not "cure" my eating disorder. I am sure they told me it would not, in those many support group meetings I attended, but I was not in any kind of a position where I could hear that and believe it. The health benefits are astounding, and the surgery was worth it just for that reason. But, as they say, "if I knew then what I know now." If I knew that I would continue to struggle and battle with my eating disorder on a daily basis, when I considered the surgery, I might have wondered "What's the point?"

THE WAR ON SUGAR

My relationship with sugar is constantly evolving and changing. The mere fact that I even have a *relationship* with sugar speaks to my eating disorder. For every person that tells you not to eat sugar and how unhealthy it is, there is another person who tells you it is OK. For every person who binges on chocolate, there is another who wolfs down potato chips, or carrot sticks, or worse. I like to eat sweet things. I find them comforting and soothing and entertaining. I am adding some other things to my life that are also comforting and soothing and entertaining, but I do not imagine that they will replace sweet things entirely.

I know a woman who has an eating disorder who went sugar free for five years. But she ate Roquefort salad dressing with a spoon right out of the jar. Another woman I know was on a food plan that was so restrictive that she would talk about "acting out" by putting two extra carrot slices on her salad. I did not want to be so obsessed with food and a food plan that it was all that I thought about. In contrast, one friend has been sugar free for over 18 months now and she speaks about how wonderful she feels and how much better her life is.

My eating disorder was constantly on the lookout for evidence that it was OK to eat sugar. I knew that there were times when I could eat sweet things rationally, and times when I could not. I wanted to find a balance. When I was upset or stressed my tendency was to turn to food. I was learning do other things, like call a friend or write in a journal or go for a walk. Yet, when I was out with friends or at a quiet, romantic dinner with my husband, I wanted to enjoy myself and sweet things were a part of that. Did I have to give that up?

Then there was all the blood sugar stuff. We probably all know by now that eating something sweet, or actually anything high in carbohydrates, will first cause your blood sugar to spike and then rapidly drop, creating more fatigue and the need for more energy. It is large amounts of any carbohydrates, not just sugar, which sets up this cycle. When I went to the diabetes nutrition classes when I was first diagnosed, they talked about limiting any particular food item to 15 grams of carbohydrates, and to not eat more than 45 grams in any one meal. Carbohydrates are not only found in sugar, but in starches, pasta, rice, potatoes, and there are even small amounts in some vegetables. An excess of *any* carbohydrate will cause that blood sugar spike and then the inevitable crash. In the classes they taught that me that I should keep my after-eating blood sugar around 160, but never over 180. When I was testing my blood sugar frequently, I discovered that oatmeal, with a little artificial sweetener on it, sent my blood sugar up to 250. And what could be healthier than oatmeal! In fact, if I ate any carbohydrates at breakfast my blood sugar would likely spike. I began to worry that all my breakfasts would have to be carbohydrate free and let us face it; carbohydrates are the easiest, quickest breakfast food items to prepare. So, when they told me in those classes that it was carbohydrates in any form, and not really the sugar, that was the culprit in that blood sugar cycle, I was relieved. Perhaps I could find a balance after all.

Is sugar a "drug?" Some people will tell you it is, and that the physiological blood sugar cycle causes "addiction." I think about it though as a process addiction rather than a substance addiction. It is not the sugar itself. It is the why and when and how much that one needs to be concerned about. This speaks also to any compulsive overeating behavior, whether it is chocolate, or Roquefort or carrots. One can binge on anything. And the woman who was sugar free for five years? Well, that did not "cure" her eating disorder or eliminate those compulsive eating behaviors. There is a part of me that kept thinking that it should have. Sometimes I believe that if I just gave up sugar, I would lose more weight and be happy. The cravings would disappear, and I would never want the demon sugar to pass my lips again.

I suspected that the reality would be different than that. Giving up sugar would not be the one and only answer to my eating disorder. First off, it set up that perfectionism thing again for me. Whenever I made a change in my life I flipped back into "from now on and forever…" Experience repeatedly told me that my eating disorder would persist through my life, and that it would vary in how dysfunctional it was. When I needed to be perfect with my eating, I became discouraged because I simply could not be. Then I felt shame and began to keep my eating behaviors secret again, and I sank quite rapidly into that hopeless and helpless abyss. My thinking would become black and white, and I would be driven to seek out the latest and greatest diet. We know how well *that* works! Emotional sobriety and food recovery would ebb and flow. As my life changed and twisted and turned, my eating disorder would twist with it.

RECOVERY – WHAT IS WORKING

It is fairly easy to find lists of coping skills and tools for recovery that involve external things. Things that you can do on the outside that effect how you think and feel on the inside. When you are stressed going for a walk might help, or writing in a journal, or calling a friend. When you feel compelled to eat something you would rather not, I have heard that brushing your teeth helps, though I have not tried that. Going to 12-step meetings helps a lot of people. Talking about their problems. Getting support from other people. Seeing a therapist. Some people find it helpful to work with a nutritionist or be on a specific food plan. Some people need psychotropic medication to help them with issues that exist alongside their eating disorder. All of these external coping skills help, and there is a lot of information out there that will list these and provide detail.

What I have focused on in this chapter are things that are *internal* that help with eating disorders and weight-loss surgery recovery. What my skills and inner resources were that I learned to draw on or change in order to be more successful in how I felt and how I lived. Sure, I did a lot of those external things, too, and they helped. But I could not just change my outsides. I had to change my insides. I could not just change my lifestyle, I had to change my thoughts and feelings and beliefs about food, about the world and about me. This is what I found that works.

MY INNER SURVIVOR

I have a strong drive for recovery. I have been through a lot in my life and have not gotten to this point without much hard work and struggle. There is a power inside me that underlies all else, my inner survivor. She has been with me my whole life and she and I have overcome some tremendous obstacles. We dealt with childhood difficulties. We got sober and off drugs. We came to terms with a debilitating depression and found a long-term solution that worked. There was my relapse back to alcohol and the subsequent four years trying to stay sober again. The eating disorder followed me everywhere. All this amongst the usual life trials of growing up, finding a meaningful career, having a family, seeing them grow up, and getting older. We have been through a lot! My survivor was always there, coaxing me on, reminding me to never give up looking for a solution, for recovery, for what would work for me. And, lo, the many times I wanted to give up! "This is too hard!" "I can't do this anymore." "You do not understand…" Yet, there was my survivor trying one more solution, reading one more book, going to one more therapy appointment, talking to one more friend. Sometimes it seemed like my inner survivor was covered up by others that were louder. In my depression, I often felt suicidal. That would get very loud at times. It was hard then to find my inner survivor. There is a part of me, way down deep inside, my very essence, which can never be destroyed. I believe that is my survivor.

As I participated in support groups, I was faced with the concept of a higher power. I often wrestled with this idea. I know they *said* that I could use my own conceptualization, but it sure sounded like they wanted me to believe in a personal "God" that somehow cared about what I did, where I lived, what job I had. I had a hard time with that idea. I might be willing to believe that there was some positive force or energy that flowed through the universe, but I did not believe in a higher power that would intervene in my life or send me checks in the mail. Perhaps my inner survivor is my higher power, evidenced by my strong drive for recovery. The getting up, over and over again, no matter how many times I fall down. Through my survivor, I can tap into that positive energy in the universe and gather the strength I need to get up again and again.

It is not easy to recover from an addiction, and often it is not fun. There are times when I would rather do *anything* other than stay in the present moment and feel my feelings. I have a strong desire to avoid my feelings, and that is a bit puzzling to me. Where along the line did I develop the belief that emotions were so scary that they had to be avoided at all costs? I must have had extraordinarily strong feelings as a child and must have had trouble dealing with them even back then. To a child, any amount of chaos can seem overwhelming. I suspect I had a stronger reaction than others to most anything, even "normal" events. And the events in my life that I believe fell outside the definition of what was "normal" played a role in my disconnecting from my feelings and experience.

That is also what alcohol and drugs did for me. They provided an internal buffer zone between the outside world and my very vulnerable insides. It was like watching my life from behind a curtain. I *looked* like I was there, in the present moment. I walked and talked like I was there, but the most vulnerable part of my essence was buried deep inside, hidden by layer upon layer of defenses. There was no question, I was scared to be in the world. I did not feel comfortable in my own skin Before alcohol and drugs, and after, my defenses were often provided by food. I could numb out using sugar, carbohydrates, any form of overeating. I was exposed to special food as a child, eating in restaurants and the like, and felt special when eating that way. It was a tremendous source of pleasure and relief.

All through this, my inner survivor persisted, sometimes quietly, sometimes more actively. My inner survivor got me through sobriety and into weight-loss surgery, with many other stops along the way. She is still with me, helping me write this book, perhaps helping you find your inner survivor. When my inner survivor connects to the positive flow of energy in the universe, I have access to a power greater than I have alone. Sanity is not engaging in addictive behaviors. The definition of insanity that I like is doing the same thing over and over again and expecting a different result. Every time I go back into overeating, believing with all my heart that "this time it will be different," I am acting insanely. Every time I start another diet believing that *this* will be different, I am acting insanely. Every time I yell at myself for how I am eating, believing that the yelling will finally cause me to change my behavior, stop overeating and lose weight, I am acting insanely. What is sane behavior for me, as far as food is concerned, is a complicated definition and has taken a long time to formulate. I have had to try out many kinds of "sanity" in order to find what would work for me. I had to experiment until I could find a way of living that I could live with.

DEFINING "SANITY"

In defining sanity for myself, I had to try a lot of insane things. There were things that seemed to work in the short term, that were not sustainable. The most notable of those was the food plan which had no sugar or flour of any kind. I did sustain that for three months. I lost 30 pounds. When I asked my husband if he noticed any difference in me, he replied, "You mean like you're not so crazy anymore?" This seemed to be THE answer to my eating disorder. I did not crave sugar; I do not even remember missing it (though I do admit to a convenient memory from time to time!). It was, however, an exceedingly difficult food plan to follow. It was way out of the mainstream of typical American eating. I was raising a family and had to make a lot of accommodations for myself. The one I remember most distinctly is when I would make spaghetti for everyone, and I would put my spaghetti sauce (with no sugar in it, of course) on a baked potato instead of on pasta like the rest of the family. My favorite breakfast became scrambled eggs on a baked potato with salsa. I do believe I have mentioned that I ate so many baked potatoes in that three months that it was three years before I could eat another one.

This food plan was too restrictive, too militant, if you will. I was not willing to sustain it. Near the end of the three months, they moved a candy machine into my work office. One day, I succumbed. Until that moment I had not realized that I had not been having sugar cravings. The minute that candy hit my system the cravings came screaming back. The food plan was over. The cravings were too intense to resist. I often think about that food plan. I often think it might be THE answer again. From time to time, I even get the book out again. I even gave it away at one point when I was in a "no more diets!" phase, only to buy it again the next time I wanted to try to force myself to "behave." If I did go back to that plan, (which I sincerely hope that I do not) I would have to modify the plan's quantities, as there was a substantial amount of food. I could not eat nearly that much at one time anymore. When I struggle the most with sugar is when the plan comes most strongly to mind. It was too difficult, however. I do not find the willingness to live within that restrictive a food plan again. The plan feeds my eating disorder if that makes sense. It sets up a "perfect" way of eating that I would not be willing to maintain. I think for me it reinforces the negative belief that I am "bad" by how I eat, and I have to be so restricted in order to be "good." I would like there to be ONE answer to this recovery business, but there is not. How I eat is only a piece of the puzzle, not the whole picture.

I tried other food plans to see if they would feel sane. I did not sustain anything for any length of time. I tried 12-step programs, to see if someone else's definition of sanity would work for me. It did not. I tried eating whatever I wanted, but that felt even less sane. My eating disorder believed that losing weight was the only sanity that was acceptable. That, however, was not happening. I even thought in writing this book that I would need to give you the answer as to how I finally lost the weight. Then you would know I had been successful. The truth, though, is that sanity for me is self-acceptance. Sanity is not shaming myself one hundred times a day for how I am eating and for how I look. It is freedom from thinking about food for hours out of every day, freedom from constantly planning what I am going to eat and when I am going to eat it. Sanity is being able to live my life happy with myself the way I am, whether I lose the weight I would like to or not.

In defining sanity, I needed a place to talk about my eating disorder and my recovery. I go to an eating disorders therapy group weekly. I have attended retreats for people who have had weight-loss surgery. I read books on eating disorders and on bariatric surgery recovery. I am writing this book. All of these activities contribute to my sanity.

JUST FOR TODAY AND ONE DECISION AT A TIME

I needed an antidote to "From now on and forever…" I needed to train my brain to stop adding "FOREVER" to every thought I had about food or exercise. Every time I had a thought or an idea about something to do with food I began to mentally add "just for today." That "forever" was so automatic that I had to purposefully catch it and change it. I decided to stop starting new diets, new programs, and new food plans – all opportunities in the past to set up that perfectionism, and then fail. I needed to break that cycle of trying to diet, following it for a few days, freaking out, giving up and then overeating again. It seemed that every time I tried to diet, I experienced a period of time after where I compensated for what I had missed by eating all my favorites, and in larger quantities than before. I kept trading the same two pounds. During the week that I was dieting I would lose two pounds. Then the week after, when I was not dieting, I would gain it back. With "just for today" I do not need to make up for what I did not eat yesterday or try to prepare for what I will eat tomorrow. Every day is its own entity. Each meal is a separate event.

I could not, however, just eat anything that I wanted, whenever I wanted it. When I did eat like that, I gained weight. I did have to pay attention to what I was eating. I had to limit my portions consciously. I thought I would be able to count on my stomach to do that for me. But, as I got farther out from the surgery, the amount of food I could eat continued to increase. As I think back, it was at about six months after the surgery that I began to be afraid that I could eat too much. It did not seem to matter how far out I was after that, or how much I could actually eat, I always thought it was too much. The doctor told me that my stomach would not stretch with the vertical sleeve surgery, but I was not sure I believed him. The fact is that I could eat enough to gain weight, regardless of whether my stomach had stretched or not. So, I had to pay attention. I began to eat about half of what I thought I wanted.

I started to be more aware of the full feeling. My eating disorder usually wanted me to finish whatever I had, whether I was full or not. I began to watch for that feeling of fullness and try to stop eating at that point. That was another good reason not to diet. When I was trying to eat a certain portion of something because it was on the plan, then I would feel compelled to eat all of it. How could I count a ½ cup of something if I only ended up eating 1/3 of it? When I was not dieting, I could stop when I felt full and not worry about how it counted.

It may sound strange, but I had to learn to throw food away. I do not remember "clean your plate" messages in my childhood, but I somehow got the value of food and learned to not be wasteful. I began to try to leave a little food left on my plate, just to practice throwing it way. I did not need to finish everything I started, but this lesson was hard won. Especially if we were talking dessert! Just recently, I was sharing a dessert and even though I got to the point of feeling sated with a few bites left, I felt compelled to finish it. I did not want more, and it was not pleasant eating more than I wanted, but I did it anyway. My eating disorder will always be with me. Learning to live with it is a daunting task. I can only manage it just for today.

Another way to combat "from now on and forever," became "one decision at a time." Instead of needing to find a way that was going to always work for me, I just had to make one decision at a time. One morning, when I stopped to buy my coffee, I chose to buy some fruit instead of some candy. That did not mean that I would always buy fruit and never buy candy again. It only counted for that one decision. Later that same day, I was driving home from work past my favorite sweet place and decided not to stop and get something for later. That did not mean that I would never stop there again. It just meant for this decision. One decision at a time, I could start to string some successes together. Since each decision was a separate event, though, I had to be careful about thinking that "success" or "failure" was cumulative. If it was cumulative then I was "good" or "bad," based on which side was accumulating, and then that perfectionism reared its ugly head again. I truly had to keep it to "One decision at a time."

"SO, WHAT'S THE PROBLEM?"

Sometimes, when things in my life are relatively smooth and calm, I wonder if I get bored. Do I have to maintain a level of drama in my life in order to feel normal? (That is a topic for another whole book right there!). There are times when I re-engage with that struggle of believing "I'm bad," and hook into the perfectionism again. Those are times I wonder if I set myself up for that struggle and maintain it simply for the sake of continuing the discomfort.

I have a really good life. My health is good, thanks to the surgery and the weight loss. I have a great husband and great kids who are developing into great adults, albeit slowly. I enjoy my career, am good at it, and am relatively financially stable (with lots of debt, like most American families). I eat a bit more than I would like to from time to time, sometimes more frequently than just "from time to time." My weight fluctuates, seemingly a bit more often in the up direction than in the down direction, though I am not sure I always have an accurate perception of that. When I take stock of all the good I have in my life, and notice that I still have an eating disorder that flares up occasionally, I sometimes have to wonder, "So, what's the problem?" In light of all the great things I have, why is it so difficult to relax and be happy? I really do not have much to complain about. What works for me is to count my blessings, as trite as that sounds, and reflect on the positive aspects of my life. When I bring to mind what is *right* with my life instead of what is *wrong,* I feel really good. I *am* happy, I enjoy what I am doing, I get along with people around me and positive energy fills me.

I can get back into that "I'm bad," though, and try to be perfect, and then the fact that I have an eating disorder seems like the end of the world. *Nothing* is right or good. I will *always* be out of control. *Everything* is miserable. I am back in black-and-white land. What *does* work is to look at all the good around me and ask myself, "SO, what's the problem?"

"I AM MORE THAN MY EATING DISORDER."

It also helps me to remember that I am more than my eating disorder. Just as being an alcoholic is no longer who I *am*, so too my eating disorder does not define me. I am a complex human being, as are we all, and there are many dimensions to my essence. There are the roles that I play – career person, wife, mother, daughter, sister, and friend. There are the activities I do – work, play, write, read, eat well (for the most part), exercise. I am an accumulation of my history and I hold a glimpse into my future. All of the events in my life have contributed to make me the person I am today. It would be foolish to think that only one aspect of who I am would define my whole being. In the throes of my eating disorder, it certainly *seems* like it defines me completely. Sometimes, food and eating seems to be all that I think about and all that I do. There are times when I get so scared about my eating that it seems like the end of the world. Those times are when I need to step back so I can see the whole picture. I need to see my family and my career, my hobbies and interests, my desires, and passions. I read parts of this book as I go along. I need to remember these things I am writing about!

PEARLS BEFORE SWINE

Recently, I had an important realization in terms of my food and my eating. I was giving myself only two options when it came to characterizing my eating – "perfect" and "bad." Again, with all-or-nothing thinking. If the food I was eating, or how much I was eating, or how often I was eating was not "perfect," then it was "bad." There was nothing in the middle, no gray. I am a visual person and I saw this represented as a coin. I was seeing only two sides of this extraordinarily complex issue.

I had to come up with a different visual characterization. I chose a pearl, and I bought myself a pearl necklace and pearl earrings to represent this. I needed to remind myself that there are MANY facets to my eating, indeed to my life that I was not allowing for in my quest for perfection. The pearl was round, not flat with only two sides. I understood that perhaps those facets of "perfect" and "bad" would still be on my pearl for a while. It might take some time before I could let them go. But I opened myself up to the possibility that there were many other facets, many other points on the pearl that represented me, with a lot of gray. There was truth and beauty and honesty. There was addiction, depression, and anxiety. There was being a mom and a wife and having a successful career. There was compassion and love and caring. All of these facets of myself fit on that small little pearl! I wore that pearl earnestly. It became my totem. Every time I touched it, I would remember that there were a lot of qualities that I possessed that were positive, in addition to the ones I found more challenging. My eating disorder did not define me, and I would not let it control me. I would find peace and serenity and true happiness in my life. They were already there. I simply had to look, and then allow myself to feel them.

This was an exceedingly difficult struggle for me. I had gotten those food messages so early, from society and the dieting industry – about how "bad" it was to eat empty calories, how "bad" it was to be overweight, how "bad" I was for gaining weight – and they seemed to be so deeply embedded as to be immovable. I had worked hard to alleviate myself of the need to be perfect in many areas of my life, but food was not one where I had been successful. Every tenth of a pound I gained, I lamented. Whoever invented digital scales anyway? Why would someone do such a thing? It was so much better in the dark ages, when you would look down at that dial from far above and would barely be able to make out whether the needle was settling at the one or the two, or at some nebulous place in between.

At the same time, I was getting messages about food being "bad" I was also learning how good it could be. Food was my best friend. It was always there; it never let me down. I could turn to it when I was lonely, sad, or scared and it would instantly calm and soothe me. I could turn to it when I was happy and celebrating and it would enhance those feelings. For me, there were times when chocolate was part of an addicted eating pattern, and times when it was not. Just as I wanted to allow gray in other areas of my life, so too did I want to allow it in terms of food. Anytime I set up a rule like "no more chocolate," it sent my inner five-year-old (remember her?) into a panic and she propelled me right to the cookie jar. The question was not so much what I was putting into my mouth, but more a question of when and why. Sure, food soothed me, but if that was the only thing that soothed me then I got into trouble with weight regain. If food was the only thing I did for fun, I struggled. If it was the only coping skill I had then my life was quite narrow in its focus. I needed to broaden my coping skills and my support system. I needed other things to do for fun and entertainment. I needed other things to soothe me. This was not to say that I would never again use food as a coping skill, but I needed other skills as well. Finding them was an important part of my journey.

MINDFUL EATING:

I practiced mindful eating when I remembered. I took small bites, chewed thoroughly, and put my fork down in between bites. I remembered to do this about half of the time. When I did remember, it helped me to sense that full feeling as soon as it hit. Then I could stop eating, most of the time. There were still times when I wanted what I was eating badly enough that I did not stop until I was overfull, and I paid for those times with discomfort.

In eating mindfully, I ate without distraction, not watching TV, or reading or doing minor tasks. I paid attention to how my food tasted, and where on my tongue I tasted it. I paid attention to color, texture, temperature, crispness or creaminess, saltiness, or sweetness. I genuinely enjoyed what I was eating when I focused on eating mindfully, and if there was something that was not an exquisite experience, I could forego it in favor of something else.

I engaged in pleasant conversation. Hot topics became off limits during family dinner time. This was a change for us. Meals were to become a time of comfort, not stress. Communication, not conflict. The temptation to try to iron out family problems was still there, as we gathered together, but we held family meetings instead for those issues and kept the family meal light and vibrant. I wanted my children to learn that eating could be a pleasant experience, a positive time shared with family and friends.

SIZE MATTERS!

Clothing size, that is! Wearing clothes that did not fit well was simply a result of my stubbornness. I would squeeze myself into those tight-fitting pants one more time, because I was darned if I were going to buy a bigger size! The problem was that I noticed that they were tight all day long, and it was a CONSTANT reminder that I was struggling with my weight yet again. Before my surgery, I had remained at the same size for over three years. All the clothes in my closet were the same size. I did not have my "skinny" clothes and my "fat" clothes. I did not like the size that I was, but it was consistent.

As I lost weight after the surgery, I got rid of clothes that became too big almost immediately. I did not want anything in my closet that was too big. I was never going to need it again! I got involved in some clothing exchanges which were tremendously helpful. Then, as my weight leveled off, so did my clothing size. I was not thrilled about where I had stopped. A friend of mine who had had the surgery about three months after I did was now a size 10, where I hovered around a 14. That did not seem exactly fair since we had lost about the same amount of weight. I had been a 2X for so long, however, that I did not mind being a Large. My mindset was such that Medium was just not even in my vocabulary.

As my weight slowly increased, it did get to the point where I had clothes that no longer fit. I was darned if I would get rid of them, however, because I was certainly going to lose the weight again! I had to get a few new things that fit me better, though, so I did not have that constant reminder that I had gained weight back. When I wore something that was too tight, I literally thought about it every minute of the day. I was so much more comfortable, both physically and emotionally, when I accepted my size right where it was, and dressed attractively and appropriately. Size does matter!

A NEW MANTRA

Another antidote to "from now on and forever" became my new mantra – "SMALL CHANGES, SLOWLY." I talked with other weight-loss surgery patients and learned what they were doing that was working or not working. I tried on ideas. Some I liked, others I discarded. A lot of people limit certain trigger foods that they are most certain to overeat. After many moons of denial, believing I could handle "just some," I began to slowly let go of some of my more pronounced trigger foods. Maybe someday they would be back, but for now I needed to stem the tide of the weight regain, and those foods were not helping. This was a SLOW, gradual process of acceptance.

I started with an "experiment" to see how I would feel if I gave up some of my favorites for just a month. About twelve days into that experiment, when I had succumbed to temptation, I saw that counting the days was another set up for me to "fail." I had to apply "just for today" to this as well. Maybe it would be a month, maybe more, maybe less. What I noticed in those twelve days was that I was not yelling at myself all day long for how I was eating. I was being gentle and allowing myself to eat what I wanted, except the triggers I was avoiding. The moment I allowed those trigger foods, I was back to yelling at myself. It might be worth letting those foods go just to be able to stop yelling at myself.

Another small change was in my support system. I started having more contact with people who had had weight-loss surgery and were dealing with the kind of issues I was dealing with. I attended weekend long retreats. I became involved in telephone coaching groups. I texted people during the day, no matter what or how I was doing. I began to stay in touch with people. I opened up and allowed myself to be honest and vulnerable. I call this one of my "small" changes, to match the mantra, but, in fact, all these changes were huge for me. To become close with people would take courage. To let go of trigger foods would take resolve and endurance. If I went without the comfort that food brought me, what would life be like? If I gave up my favorite form of fun and entertainment, would I be bored? Would I be boring? If I dropped some of my defenses, would people accept me? These were all fears I had that generated anxiety that I then ate over. The cycle had to stop. And it began to change, slowly.

SEMANTICS AND VOCABULARY

"Could" rather than "Should": Semantics are important. Certain words feel differently when you say them. One important change in my vocabulary that helped a lot was replacing the word "should" with the word "could." "Should" activated all my shame. I should eat this way. I should feel this way. I should weigh this amount. I should exercise. By saying

"should" it, first of all, implied that I was not doing those things. Another implication was that I was "bad" if I did not do what I "should." Replacing the word "should" with the word "could" changes the entire meaning, I *could* eat this way – in other words, I have a choice. I *could* exercise. No judgment implied if I do not.

"Good" "Bad" "Right" "Wrong" (GBRW): Four words I tried to eliminate from my vocabulary. I was constantly thinking of food as "good, bad, right or wrong." This led to thinking of myself as "good, bad, right or wrong." That led to perfectionism, which led to shame, which led to more GBRW. My eating disorder was not GBRW, and I was not GBRW for having one. My eating was not GBRW, my weight gain was not GBRW. All these things just were what they were. When I did not judge them, the shame let up a bit, and I experienced a more peaceful feeling.

AFFIRMATIONS

Saying affirmations is hokey and dumb. I do not like doing it. The problem is that it works! When I tell myself positive things about myself repeatedly, I end up believing them. It is the old self-fulfilling prophecy idea – if you tell a child s/he is stupid often enough they will eventually believe you and that will affect their academic performance. Well, it turns out, if you tell someone (even yourself) that they are good often enough they will eventually believe that too!

When my therapist first suggested I say affirmations, despite what I thought about them, I was so depressed that I was desperate. I would have flown to the moon if it would have helped at that point. I did not like the whole idea of affirmations, but I was willing to do just about anything. As I used them more, I generally found that after about three weeks of saying an affirmation I would actually notice a difference in how I felt and what I thought. Saying affirmations was certainly a small price to pay for feeling so much better!

When I remembered to do them, I started with some basic ones and I repeated them out loud several times each. I often did this when I was driving, or when I was walking from one building to another at work. The ones I started with were:

> "I am worthwhile, and I am good."
>
> "I am important, and I matter."
>
> "I am growing and changing."
>
> "I love and accept myself today exactly as I am."
>
> "Other people love and accept me today exactly as I am."
>
> "I am OK no matter what I eat or what I weigh."
>
> "I make appropriate food choices based on my goals."

The first two were quite simple and scripted to reach the younger part of myself that thought she was eternally "bad." Others appealed to an older part of myself, including my adult, and would lead me into right action. I would use the last one when I was ordering in a restaurant, or when I wanted something that I could really live without. Because I *am* OK no matter what I eat or weigh, AND I still want to make appropriate food choices based on my goals.

Another set of affirmations I developed was a bit more general, as I was attempting to take my focus off of doing the "right" thing with food even in my affirmations! One day, when I was having a particularly difficult time of it, I scripted these new affirmations and began saying them in earnest. I said them several times every day. These affirmations were:

> "I am great the way I am."
>
> "I feel good about myself."
>
> "My mind is peaceful and untroubled."
>
> "I am happy and healthy."
>
> "I am finding my own recovery."
>
> "I feel safe in the world."
>
> "The universe surrounds me with healing energy and love."

The happy and healthy one was significant because when I was scripting it, I got in touch with gratitude that the surgery had improved my health. As I said earlier, the fact that my health would improve was not really why I wanted to have the surgery. And to be honest, I was beginning to wonder if I would have had the surgery, if I had known how tough it was going to be to adjust. But just in that moment of self-doubt, a sense of peace and gratitude settled over me, perhaps for the first time. I *was* glad I had had the surgery, and I *would* do it again, even knowing what I know now.

CEASE FIRE

My eating disorder had many war-like characteristics and I often felt like I was engaged in battle. Which side would win – the eating disorder or recovery? The one I fed the most. In truth, there would be no final winning or losing, there is only the journey. I live "in recovery." I do not consider myself "recovered" from my eating disorder. As much as I hated having an eating disorder, as much as I wanted to go through life eating whatever I wanted with no consequences (there was that 5-yr-old again!), in reality – no one gets to do that. I could say I wanted to be like a "normal" eater, but it would be difficult to define what that is. I think it is "normal" in our society to worry about your weight, to drift from one diet to another, to be persistently trying to achieve some ideal model of attractiveness. I do not think that men are immune from this, but I do think the trend is stronger among women. So, I am in good company.

Relief from an eating disorder is hard won. It takes effort and diligence. One cannot rest in recovery, at least not for awfully long. All of the tools I have discussed help. Some of them help a lot, most of the time. Others help some, some of the time.

They help much more when I remember to use them! I want to believe, no, to *remember*, that my weight-loss surgery has been successful. My serious health issues are resolved. I can go hiking with my husband. I can swim with my Labrador.

Just for today, one decision at a time, I declared a cease-fire. I may not have been able to win the war, once and for all, but I could stop the battle. I just did not want to fight myself anymore. For that is what was really happening. No one else was telling me what to eat, or how to be. The shame that yelled at me all day long was generated by old hurts. The perfectionism that was the perceived solution to that shame was internal. There needed to be an end to my fear of gaining all my weight back, an end to the seemingly constant negative thoughts and obsessions about myself and about food. I was missing out on the life that was blossoming right in front of me! I needed to find other ways to comfort and soothe myself. Most of those were internal as well. The way I talked to myself (no more yelling!), the way I thought about my life ("So, what's the problem?" and "I am more than my eating disorder") and connecting with important support people all helped me find the peacefulness that I desired.

YOUR JOURNEY

If we use the term "eating disorder" loosely and do not worry about the clinical definition, I think it is safe to say that anyone overweight enough to consider and qualify for bariatric surgery has an "eating disorder." Just because someone does not meet the clinical definition does not mean they do not suffer. The question is, "Will the eating disorder go away if I have the surgery?" The answer is "No." I really wanted it to, and I really thought it would, but it did not.

Perhaps you are reading this book because you too have an eating disorder that was not "cured" by weight-loss surgery. Perhaps you are considering weight-loss surgery and are reading everything you can get your hands on. Perhaps you have an eating disorder and are wondering if weight-loss surgery will be your answer. I hope that this may also be an instructional book in the world of the medical community.

I hope I have painted a somewhat more realistic, psychological picture of life after weight-loss surgery than you might get from the doctor's office. Historically, the medical profession has believed in weight-loss surgery and touted its benefits. They have not often, though, understood the emotional upheaval it causes and the adjustments that must be made. They like to say, "I operated on your stomach, not your brain," when confronted with their lack of understanding. The conscientious doctors will have some sort of support system in place for after surgery that may, or may not, be helpful. In the end, though, it is a personal, individual journey and you have to find your own way.

I encourage you to look beyond your eating disorder and see the big picture that is your whole life. Enjoy the honeymoon period and the initial rapid weight loss. Soak up the compliments and the admiration, you will need them later. When the high starts to subside, and your hunger starts to return, take some of the suggestions in this book and work with them. Use "Just for today," and see that you are more than your eating disorder. Get some sort of therapy to guide you through the adjustment, preferably with someone who understands eating disorders. Find a relationship with food that works for you, that you can and are willing to live with. And, for heaven's sake, understand that your relationship with food will evolve and change. Nothing is set in stone, and no decision is irreversible. Write a mantra for yourself that is loving and caring and consider using affirmations to smooth over some of those rough spots. Discover a meaningful totem, like the pearl is for me. Lastly, find your inner survivor, the part of you that persists tenaciously. Introduce her to your inner 5-yr-old (and any other ages you find in there!) and start working together to move toward your goals. Whether you have more weight to lose, are struggling emotionally or simply want to find a more peaceful relationship with food and with yourself, you can find your way. Get support. You do not have to do this alone. Let us find our way on this road together. All you have to do is to be willing, and to begin.

EPILOGUE

A year ago, when I started writing this book, I was in a much different place than I am now. My journey through this writing has been a transformative experience. It has compelled me to look at my story from the inside out. I went back to places from my childhood that I had not been to in a long time. It even brought me to a place of looking at the world through my parents' eyes and seeing what their world was like as I was being raised. Our American culture has always placed a premium on attractiveness and beauty, and has endlessly linked this with physical appearance, especially body size. We all contend with these lofty ideals and unreasonable standards every day. Fortunately, in my daughter's generation there have been some incredibly positive role models in the fashion and entertainment industry, women who are of larger size. I grew up with "Twiggy." My daughter grew up with Queen Latifah, Roseanne Barr, Oprah. As I wrote, I found myself continuing to struggle with my weight and that diet mentality. Every time the shame of gaining weight overcame me, I would rush back to this book and re-read "What is Working." I would have to remind myself that I had said I would not go on diets anymore, that they set up an unrealistic goal of perfectionism for me. Those were black-and-white traps. I had to stay out of their snare. Once, as I was editing, I got through the entire book up through "What's Not Working," but I stopped there, due to time constraints. Well, that catapulted me into a major depression, because I had only read about the problem and had not gotten to the solution!

I had to come up with a way of living I could live with, and this book played a tremendous role in that journey. A journey that will continue, despite my desire to have all this figured out from now on and forever. I could not ignore my eating disorder, but I did not want it to be the main focus of my life either. I *am* more than my eating disorder and the more I focus on the positive other things I do and am, the better I feel.

My understanding of myself and my eating disorder continues to evolve. Some days I think it is a good idea to have at least a little structure to my eating, and other days not. What I really want is freedom from worrying all the time. Worrying about my weight, about what I put in my mouth. How many calories does it have? Carbohydrates? Fat grams? If I ride my stationary bike for five extra minutes, how many calories do I burn? What can I eat when I go to this party? Do I bring my own food? Do I cook differently for my family than I do for myself? STOP! My eating disorder makes me crazy! I wanted recovery, to have my mind be at peace, and this book gave me as many good ideas to help me achieve that as I hope it has given you.

What would recovery from my eating disorder look like? I am not completely sure yet, but I know it will not include searching and hopping from one diet to the next. I want recovery to be an acceptance of who I am no matter what I weigh or what I look like. I am coming into the aging time of life and will have to find many pockets of self-confidence and self-acceptance as the years go on. The pounds would have to come off, if they were going to, through lifestyle changes and eating less overall, without trying to fit that "eating less" into someone else's definition. Working with my nutritionist I increased my fruit and vegetable intake, decreased my starch and sugar intake, and closely watched my protein. Those small changes slowly would have to be enough. They were not enough for my eating disorder, and my weight continued to fluctuate, up a few pounds and then down a few pounds, but the upward trend seemed to have slowed or stopped. I had become conscious of the problem and frightened of the consequences of not doing anything.

My heart and soul are in this book and in the ideas that you find here. Some you may find helpful, others not. I only ask that you pay attention – to your recovery, to your health, and to yourself. You will find your way as I have found mine, just for today and one decision at a time.

CPSIA information can be obtained
at www.ICGtesting.com
Printed in the USA
LVHW032010220323
742311LV00014B/1204

9 781647 195939